What Practitioners Are Saying about This Book

After reading your book for the third time, studying your video course, and listening to the cassette tapes, I have incorporated your techniques into my sessions without hesitation. When I added your library technique, it made a world of a difference to the success of my clients. I truly believe the library technique is the best therapy that I have ever used. And your testing after the library is just brilliant; this alone has skyrocketed my success.

After studying with other well know therapists, Otto, Churchill, Motton, Kein and Krasner, you are the only one who ever gave a true definition of hypnosis. When I teach classes I follow and use your teachings as the correct definition.

As a dedicated student of the Preston method I would like to know if there is a way of receiving a certificate from you so that I may display it on my office wall. If a test is needed to be written or whatever, please let me know.

I thank you for the knowledge and expertise in the field of hypnosis and thank you for sharing this with the world.

Alex Szwed
alexszwed@allstream.net
www.journeyofthemind.com

HYPNOSIS: MEDICINE OF THE MIND

DISCLAIMER

Since the success or failure of any therapy depends upon many unknown factors, it is almost impossible to ascertain (within a reasonable degree of certainty) what response any individual may exhibit during the hypnotic session. Hypnotherapy is not a medical procedure, nor is it the practice of medicine. No hypnotherapist should guarantee the anticipated response or result of a hypnotic session.

HYPNOSIS: MEDICINE OF THE MIND

OF THE MIND

A Complete Manual
on Hypnosis for the
Beginner, Intermediate,
and Advanced Practitioner

MICHAEL D. PRESTON,
J.D., PH.D.

Tiger Maple Press
Tempe, Arizona

Tiger Maple Press
A Division of Dandelion Enterprises, Inc.
Tempe, Arizona

Library of Congress Cataloging-in-Publication Data
Preston, Michael D.
Hypnosis: medicine of the mind – a complete manual on hypnosis for the
beginner, intermediate and advanced practitioner

Library of Congress Catalog Card Number 2005907170
ISBN 0-963294-74-1
3rd Edition, by Tiger Maple Press
2nd Edition, published by Ulyssian Publications, 2001, ISBN 1-930580-11-8
1st Edition by Michael D. Preston, 1998

Cover and Book Revisions by TJ Publish, www.tjpublish.com

CONTENTS

INTRODUCTION

Hypnotism is the science of communication and concentration utilizing the thought process of the individual. The mind, consisting of the conscious and the subconscious, is employed to remove the difficulties, symptoms, and suffering. It is absolutely necessary in the treatment to utilize the beneficial powers of the mind to search and recall all experiences causing the person's problems. The amazing power of the human mind enables it to accurately recall these experiences while in a deep state of hypnosis. As the patient recalls the true facts in the development of the disease, he achieves intellectual clarity about the origin of his problem and then creates suggestions of his own that often lead to successful removal of his difficulties.

The hypnotist cannot control the patient's will but can only aid by directing the patient's thought process to develop beneficial suggestions. Nothing can, or will, be done until and unless there is full cooperation on behalf of the subject. Lacking the full cooperation, the hypnotic session is doomed to failure.

There is no safer medical modality than hypnosis, but unfortunately, those who need the treatment most are likely to reject it due to their failure to understand the real meaning of hypnosis. This book should alleviate those fears, and bring them health and happiness.

Hypnosis is a change of consciousness. The subconscious mind contains links to other conscious entities in the universe. This connecting link provides the basis for understanding in detail, paranormal phenomena, including "mind over matter."

This is to say that there is one mind, one intelligence, and one presence in the entire universe.

1

THE HISTORY OF HYPNOSIS

Hypnosis began with the advent of mankind. In subsequent chapters, hypnosis and its conditions and benefits will be discussed. However, for the purposes of historical matters, let's begin with man's use of hypnosis.

Virtually, all early and primitive people performed special rituals and ceremonies as part of their everyday lives. An integral part of these rites included monotonous beating of the drums, rhythmic chanting, and dancing. Individuals dressed in various garments denoting their status in the community; healers and witch doctors were revered for having special or supernatural powers. The continuous chanting, dancing, and participation in the ceremony and ritual brought about a heightened response in the participants which, in turn, led to the realization of their expectancies. The early belief was that if a person participated in the rituals or if the ceremonies were done for and on his behalf, he would benefit from the expected results of the ritual. It was immaterial whether or not these rituals were religious, spiritual, or healing ceremonies, as the expected result was affected by the participation and belief.

So from the beginning of time and before history was recorded, two essential elements of hypnosis were established: (1) the expectancy of the result and (2) the conviction that the result would occur. In the tenth century, Avicenna, the great physician, observed: "The imagination can fascinate and modify the man's body, making him ill or restoring him to health." As early as 1500 B.C., the Ebers Papyrus recorded a treatment in which a physician, while uttering strange chantings, merely laid his hands on the head or body of the patient and these chantings effected a cure in the afflicted person.

The Egyptians continued to practice healing, and word of their success eventually spread far and wide throughout the adjoining lands, as far away as England and Asia Minor. As a symbol and physical evidence of their beliefs, the Egyptians built various temples in which the priests practiced their "suggestions," "rituals," and "cures" in the treatment of those afflicted and suffering.

Franz Anton Mesmer was born on May 23, 1734, in Austria and received his Doctor of Medicine degree in 1766. Mesmer became acquainted with the theories of hypnotism and incorporated his knowledge into his medical practice, attempting to cure his patients' symptoms and difficulties. However, his lack of experience in hypnotism and his inability to gain additional knowledge of the art led him to consider the phenomenon of hypnotism as having its origin in some magnetic field. Mesmer described his "animal magnetism" as follows:

1. Animal magnetism is a universal fluid consisting of an absolute plenum in nature and the medium of all mutual influences between the celestial bodies and betwixt the earth and animal bodies.
2. It is the most subtle fluid in nature, capable of flux, reflux, and of receiving, propagating, and continuing all kinds of motion.
3. The animal body is subjected to the influences of this fluid by means of the nerves, which are immediately affected by it.
4. The human body has poles and other properties analogous to the magnet.
5. The action and virtue of animal magnetism may be communicated from one body to another, whether animate or inanimate.
6. It operates at a great distance without the intervention of any body.

7. It is increased and reflected by mirrors, communicated, propagated and increased by sound, and may be accumulated, concentrated, and transported.
8. Notwithstanding the universality of this fluid, all animal bodies are not affected by it; on the other hand, there are some animal bodies (though few in number) the presence of which destroys all effects of animal magnetism.
9. That by means of this fluid, nervous diseases are cured immediately and others mediately ... and its virtues, in fact, extend to the universal cure and preservation of mankind.

Sometime around 1777, Mesmer treated a blind pianist, Maria Teresa Paradis, and following his treatments, her sight was restored. All previous attempts by other physicians had failed. Mesmer's success continued to grow until 1784 when, after lengthy investigation, his animal magnetism was labeled a fraud. Following this, Mesmer moved to Switzerland where he died in 1815. The terms "mesmerized" and "mesmerism" evolved from his name.

Dr. James Braid, an English physician, became interested in hypnotism somewhere around 1841 when he attended a lecture given by a Frenchman named LaFontaine, who demonstrated some of Mesmer's techniques. Following this demonstration, Dr. Braid began a detailed study of hypnotism and in the process developed several of his own induction techniques.

For several years, Dr. Braid conducted various experiments with his patients. He subsequently renamed mesmerism "hypnotism" after the Greek word *hypnos*, meaning "sleep." Later, Dr. Braid realized that hypnotism was not a form of sleep but a deep state of concentration of the mind. He tried to rename hypnosis, but the word was so entrenched, eventually he abandoned his efforts to effect a change. Consequently, the name remains today, giving the general public the false impression that the subject is in a deep sleep. This fallacy is perpetuated by those hypnotists who continue to use the word without explaining what we, as hypnotists, mean by its term.

One of the least known practitioners and one who probably contributed the most to medical hypnosis is Dr. James Esdaile. Dr. Esdaile, like Dr. Braid, an English physician, studied medicine in Edinburgh, where he graduated in 1830. Sometime later, he obtained a position with the East India Company and set up practice in Calcutta, India, where he remained most of his life. He was a man of extreme medical intelligence and probably performed more surgical operations with the use of hypnosis as an anesthetic than any other surgeon up to the present time. By the end of 1845, he had more than a hundred major operations to his credit with the use of hypnosis. After receiving many favorable reports on his medical endeavors, the governor of India placed Dr. Esdaile in charge of a small hospital outside Calcutta, where he could continue his experimental operations with the use of hypnosis. By the end of his first year at that hospital, he had more than 135 major operations to his credit. As is to be expected, he was criticized by some of his colleagues. In spite of these criticisms, his fame continued to spread and by the time he left India, he had performed thousands of operations with the use of hypnosis. In the years following his departure from India, Dr. Esdaile wrote articles criticizing the medical profession for not accepting hypnosis as a real medical tool. He finally took his case to the general public to convince them of the true benefits in the field of medical cures for such ailments as palsy, sciatica, lumbago, convulsions, and other serious symptomatic problems. His greatest contribution was in promoting the value of hypnosis in creating anesthesia and analgesia.

Dr. A. A. Liebault received his medical degree in 1850 and continued to maintain a country practice that kept him quite busy. His practice in hypnotism was gratuitous and because of this, he gained the respect of the patients and others who knew him. He had started to experiment with the use of hypnosis at an early age and quite some time before he earned his medical degree. He continued his studies after his graduation, keeping a close record of his results. It wasn't long thereafter that he conceived the idea that all of the phenomenon of hypnosis were subjective in origin. Dr. Liebault was the first physician to conclude this and wrote a book on hypnotism which took him two years to publish. This book contained detailed information on his hypnotic therapeutic sessions and the fascinating results.

Dr. Eugene Azam was on the faculty of medicine at Bordeaux as a correspondent for the Academy of Medicine in Paris. Dr. Azam's contribution to the advancement of hypnosis is in his discovery of the splitting of the conscious. It was he who made medical practitioners aware of two levels of awareness. These two levels of awareness are now referred to as the conscious and subconscious. He endeavored to attribute the phenomena of hypnosis to the psychiatric influence of suggestion rather than the influence of magnetism as had been so popular with previous practitioners.

Probably one of the most noted doctors to be influenced by the field of hypnotism was Dr. Sigmund Freud. To fully set forth and understand his influence would take more than the time and space allotted here. Many books have been written on his works and they only begin to cover his entire contribution to the field of psychiatry. Although Dr. Freud used words and techniques related to hypnosis, such as suggestion of relaxation and extensive use of imagination together with the touching of the forehead or visual concentration, he preferred to use the term "psychoanalysis" rather than "direct suggestion."

Dr. Freud studied hypnotism with Dr. Hippolite Berhmeim and Dr. Jean Martin Charcot. It was Dr. Charcot's belief that in order to be hypnotized, one must be of weak mind. This fallacy even persists today even though there have been so many books written on the subject. Dr. Charcot further influenced Dr. Freud because he persisted in maintaining the position that hypnosis was a sign of weakness and of a nervous disposition. Dr. Freud eventually abandoned hypnosis because he was embarrassed by the lack of his ability to obtain a deep state of hypnosis in his patients and because the cures he was able to obtain were only temporary, since his posthypnotic suggestions could not be maintained.

In 1955, the British Medical Association gave its unqualified approval of hypnosis, instructing the Council on Medical Health to investigate the value of hypnosis in medicine. At the June 1958 meeting of the American Medical Association, hypnosis was approved as a medical tool without a dissenting vote.

During the past thirty years or more, many physicians, dentists, psychiatrists, psychologists, social workers, and nonlicensed persons have taken up the cause of hypnosis, thereby educating the general public as to its therapeutic values and benefits.

Credit for continuous contributions in the use of hypnosis should be given to such professionals as Dr. Lewis R. Wolberg; Dr. William J. Bryan, Jr; Dr. S. J. Van Pelt; Dr. Milton H. Erickson; and others. However, we should not take lightly the valuable contributions of such non-professionals as Leslie M. LeCron, Harry Arons, Edward Barons, and Dave Elman, just to name a few.

From this brief history of hypnosis, it can now be said without contradiction that the following principles of hypnosis have been established:

1. Hypnosis is not animal magnetism or a universal fluid.
2. Hypnosis is not a form of sleep.
3. The consciousness of a person can be, and is, split into a conscious and a subconscious.
4. The recalling of a traumatic experience or event can be utilized to remove the symptom.
5. Hypnosis can be used in dealing with the cause of the symptom as well as removal of the symptom.
6. The phenomenon of hypnosis is subjective in origin.
7. Hypnosis is a science in itself.

8. Hypnosis is a valuable tool in the treatment of symptomatic conditions.
9. Hypnosis has a place in the medical field.

2

DEFINITION OF HYPNOSIS

Webster's New Collegiate Dictionary defines hypnosis as: "a state that resembles sleep that is induced by a hypnotizer whose suggestions are easily and readily accepted by the person." Webster further defines hypnosis as "a sleep-inducing agent." However, practitioners agree that Webster's definition is entirely wrong. Hypnosis is not a sleep-like condition. As a matter of fact, the subject becomes more alert as the session continues. Many assume that just because the subject's eyes are closed, the person is asleep. Furthermore, since the word "sleep" is so frequently used in the induction procedure, confusion between physical sleep and hypnosis has persisted.

I recently attended a convention in Las Vegas and asked the five persons sitting on a panel for their definition of hypnosis. I promptly received five different answers. Even those who have been using, studying, and teaching hypnosis cannot agree on a simple definition.

The main stumbling block in defining hypnosis is the interpretation of the words we use to define it. We all have different interpretations of the meaning of certain words; so if we cannot agree to the meaning, we have a difficult time agreeing on a definition. However, the reason we have so many different definitions is not that the practitioners do not have knowledge of the subject of hypnosis. It is primarily due to their experiences in utilizing the phenomena as well as the differences in their own personalities.

Hypnosis, like all other sciences, has its origin in mystery and superstition, and time has been very slow in removing the evils associated with its origin. In the past, hypnosis has gone through periods and cycles of acceptance and rejection – a period of acceptance being followed by generations of rejection. It must be recognized that at no time did hypnosis or its prior forms ever completely cease to exist. From the beginning of mankind to the present time, it has been used in various forms for ages.

Since the practice of the art of hypnosis has extended over such a long period of time, the people living in earlier periods had a different conception of hypnosis than those of more recent times. Consequently, the acceptance of hypnosis has greatly suffered because of the poor definition of hypnosis. Mesmer described the phenomenon as a form of magnetism. Brownell described hypnotism as having its origin in mesmerism. Dr. Milton Kline described the hypnotic phenomenon as "being in a state of emotional readiness, or perhaps emotional responsiveness when a subject is sent into action." Dr. Charcot described it as a "disease." Dr. Albert Moll described hypnosis: "If we take a pathological condition of the organism as necessary for hypnosis, we shall be obliged to conclude that nearly everyone is not quite right in the head." Leslie M. LeCron stated that to most people the word "hypnotism" conveys a suggestion of the supernatural. The mental image of hypnotism brings immediate visions of a sinister person with glittering and piercing eyes. Dr. Milton H. Erickson had devoted many chapters to definitions, yet he defined everything but hypnosis.

Most people who have attempted to define hypnosis have defined the end result of that state or condition as opposed to the state or condition itself. As Dr. Albert Mall said, "Hypnotism consists of a voluntary submission of a patient to a series of carefully controlled suggestions whose purpose is to increase the suggestibility of submission so the specific therapeutic suggestions may be accepted." Some consider hypnosis as being a semi-aware state, such as going in and out of or drifting many times in consciousness during the day as we do when we're daydreaming. Some consider it a flight into fantasy; for example, we're neither here nor there. J. H. Eysenk explained hypnosis as the ability of an individual to direct the whole force of nervous energy into a small number of nervous channels, thereby reducing the synaptic resistance and facilitating the passage of nervous energy. Dr. Heinz Hammerschlaug defined hypnosis as waking suggestion and noted that hypnosis in and of itself does not characterize different states of consciousness in the subject, but only the variations in his outer behavior.

On the other hand, we must point out that a state of hypnosis exists when the subject's state of awareness undergoes a definite change. Dr. Lewis K. Boswell considers hypnosis an unusual state in which the mind is so completely focused on the immediate thoughts or events that it disregards all surrounding stimuli. During this unusual state, the mind is capable of accepting helpful suggestions in a manner far exceeding its normal capacity; hence it is possible to quickly and effectively recall any significant conditions and events. Dr. William J. Bryan, Jr., defines hypnosis as an altered state of consciousness, similar to but not the same as being awake, similar to but not the same as being asleep, produced by a presence of two conditions: (1) the central focus of attention and (2) the surrounding area of inhibition.

The definition used by most persons for hypnosis is: "an altered state of consciousness." Some will go so far as to say it is a trance state of consciousness; others say it is a state of super-awareness.

Probably the best way to approach the definition of hypnosis is by the process of elimination. So let's eliminate those descriptions that we now know it *isn't* and see what's left.

First, it should be emphasized that hypnosis is not a trance, state of sleep, or unconsciousness.

Consider for the moment that a trance state is one in which the individual is not in full and complete control of all of his physical and mental capacities. A hypnotized person is not in a trance. One under the influence of intoxicants or drugs may be in a trance, depending upon the amount of drugs or alcohol that had been consumed. The more consumed, the deeper the trance state. One's physical faculties have been impeded by the nature and amount of the drug.

Nor is one in a state of hypnosis like a zombie – that is, unable to formulate any thought or coordinated movement. Here particularly, a person can readily be confused in the definition of hypnosis by what it does and not what it is. A person in a state of hypnosis can, by accepting suggestions, respond in a manner so as to appear to be confused or in a trance. Under proper suggestions, a subject can be made to suffer temporary amnesia. Analgesia can be made to appear in the subject so that he is unable to feel his extremities. One's speech may be entirely inhibited by proper suggestion in hypnosis. All of these are the end result of proper suggestions while in a state of hypnosis.

Several years ago, about ten o'clock in the evening, after having completed twelve hours of continuous sessions, I was waiting to have my sandwich served to me when a young fellow came over and stated he knew something about hypnosis. He went on to explain that he thought his subconscious mind was not as strong as his conscious mind and that there was no such thing as hypnosis. Within thirty seconds and before he realized it, he was in a deep state of hypnosis. I then suggested that his feet were glued to the floor and he couldn't walk back to his table, and when I permitted him to return to the table, he wouldn't be able to take a second drink from any glass. When I asked him to return to his table, he was unable to walk and looked at me in utter amazement. I then suggested that he could walk back to his table, which he promptly did. However, after taking one drink from his water glass, he couldn't lift the glass off the table. He tried in vain to lift the glass, but it wouldn't come off the table, although everyone else at the table had no difficulty in lifting the glass. Another glass of water was brought over to him and he proceeded to drink from it. After one drink, he couldn't lift the second glass. Everyone kept lifting the glasses and started to tease him for being a weakling who couldn't even lift a little glass for a second drink. Try as he would, he failed. Little did he recognize that during all of this time, he was deeply hypnotized. When I finished eating, I stopped at his table and removed the suggestions. He promptly apologized for speaking so rudely about a subject he knew very little about.

I usually try to stay away from this type of situation as it tends to convey the general impression that the hypnotist controls the subject. This young gentleman was not in a trance and knew at all times just what he was doing and was aware of his surrounding circumstances. The condition of his inability to lift the glass was created by suggestion.

Webster's New Collegiate Dictionary defines sleep as "a natural periodic suspension of consciousness during which the powers of the body are restored," and "a state marked by a diminution of feeling." We normally recognize the state of sleep as when one is not aware of surroundings, conditions, and circumstances as in a state of being unconscious.

One of the most widely known and common misconceptions is that when one is hypnotized, consciousness is lost. Due to this misconception, persons who need and desire hypnosis fail to utilize its benefits. This misconception impairs their confidence and makes it more difficult for the subject to obtain the necessary or desired results. At every level of hypnosis, even the deepest state possible, the person being hypnotized is always completely aware of all his surrounding circumstances. At no time is the person unaware. The greater the depth, the more awareness, and the better the results. There is an increased attention to the hypnotist's suggestions. One of the greatest difficulties the hypnotist will encounter is to convince the subject that he has been hypnotized. Over 90 percent of all people hypnotized for the first time will deny they have been hypnotized and assert as the reason they were not, that they were entirely aware of everything said and done during the session. To remove this problem, it is important that the hypnotist assures in advance that the subject will always be aware and cognitive during the session. Even then, the problem of convincing the subject will arise.

The word "sleep" is normally associated with the condition we experience in the evening when we lie in bed with our eyes closed, unaware of what is about us. Confusion is produced by the operator's suggestions that "you are going deep, deep, deep, asleep." The better practice is to refrain from using the word "sleep" until after the deepening processes have been completed and it's time for the therapy or suggestions. You will notice in subsequent chapters where the verbalization is done that the words "relax" and "relaxation" are used in place of "sleep." The word "sleep" is not introduced until its meaning has been fully and completely explained.

Hypnosis, in my opinion, is not an altered state of consciousness or awareness. Here we must again come to grips with our endeavors to be precise with our interpretations of words. The word "altered" can have several meanings. It can mean changed, modified, amended, remodeled, made different, or have any other meaning that one might feasibly desire. If we have an altered state of consciousness, then how many states do we have? Is there more than one degree of change in each state, such as mild, light, medium, and deep? Who then makes this change, the hypnotist or the subject? If we alter the state into a different state, then in what state was the subject before the change? The definition leads to more questions than we have answers for. It may appear paradoxical that in striving to be precise about our use of words, we become vague in attempting to define hypnosis. Many books and articles have been written on hypnosis without coming to grips with the question of precisely just what they are writing about. Many writers and investigators have been quite willing to admit that a meaningful definition has eluded them.

Before we proceed further with the definition of hypnosis, let us review some of the characteristics and makeup of the human being that history, experiments, and investigations have taught us. We all recognize that during the daytime, when we are up and about, we utilize our senses, such as sight and hearing, and recognize those things making up our close surroundings and environment. In other words, we are conscious of our surroundings. Consciousness means awareness. What we see and hear are not momentary passing impressions. At some future time, we can recall seeing and hearing certain things. Some events we can immediately recall, some we recall after considerable deliberation, and others we are unable to recall at all. Experience has taught us that we gather information by the use of our senses: sight, hearing, smell, feel, and taste. Since these experiences or events can be recalled at some future date, they must have been stored somewhere for future use. The chapter on the brain in this book explains the method by which this information is stored in the brain.

Each of the nerve cells (neurons) consists of a cell body containing a nucleus, a long fiber (axon), and varying numbers of smaller fibers called dendrites. These dendrites have receptors on their surface. The function of the receptors is to receive chemical messages from nearby neurons. Each receptor receives only one message, always the same message. The incoming message fits into the receptors, resembling a key into a lock: same key, same lock. Upon receiving the message, it is then passed onward which, in turn, causes cells, glands, and tissues to respond in accordance with the original message. This nerve impulse is conveyed from the nerve body out along the axon, where it terminates on other varying numbers of other cell bodies or other nerves. This is the means of conveying an impulse or impression from one part of the body to another. Each of the billions of neurons in the human brain may have over a thousand synapses (points of contact between nerve cells). Some nerve cells in the cortex may have as many as 200,000 connections. Consider for a moment that as many as tens of thousands of impressions, impulses, and events are being conveyed simultaneously. Through the use of our consciousness, such things as awareness, facts, events, impulses, and impressions are gathered and stored in the cortex while others maintain that the entire brain is the recipient.

For our purposes, let's consider the brain as the storage area or memory bank. When a person is asked a question for which the answer requires some concentration or thought, a whole new process of awareness becomes evident. A simple experiment is to ask someone a question that requires some thought. You will notice the person will close the eyelids or look away in some direction or focus their attention on some spot while searching for the answer. When the answer is secured, then the person will focus his eyes and state the answer recalled.

Dr. Eugene Azam recognized many years ago that there was a splitting of the consciousness. Every able practitioner of hypnosis recognizes that in hypnosis a person can recall events not available in the ordinary waking state. This second state of conscious awareness is usually called the subconsciousness. Some refer to it as superconsciousness, while others prefer preconsciousness.

Nowhere in the entire anatomy of the body and brain is there a cell, gland, or material matter called consciousness. Consciousness is not a material thing. It occupies no space. It has no essence. We are dealing with something that cannot be seen or touched. It is spirit in form. Yet we have the conscious and the subconscious, the outer awareness and the inner awareness.

The function of the outer awareness, consciousness, is to gather information, impulses, and impressions from those elements and happenings around us, and send this information into the brain for storage and future reference. However, on the conscious level, before this information is stored in the memory bank, it is filtered, analyzed, and sorted. Every experience, event, idea, need, desire, and emotion such as hate, love, pain, or joy are registered and stored in the brain cells to remain forever, unless actively removed. The greater the thought given to the emotion or event, the greater the future impact. The more credible, the greater the response. The more acceptance is attached to the event or impulse, the quicker the response. It is much easier to recall important and believable events than those of little or no importance. Burn your hand once on a hot stove and the next time you begin to be aware of the heat, there is an instant retreat. It is much easier to recall the events of your wedding than those of a friend's wedding which you attended.

The subconscious mind or subconscious awareness has the ability to function in conjunction with the conscious mind and yet independently. Remember there are thousands of impulses and impressions operating simultaneously that must be processed through the conscious and subconscious awareness.

Imagine a person walking on the sidewalk, listening to the radio he is carrying, eating a candy bar, and watching the parade march down the street. Each color, horizontal or vertical line, curve, and distance are being processed from the eyes through the thousands of nerve cells into the brain for reassembly to create a picture in the brain. Every sound, every pitch – high, low, and in between – are also being sent through the nerves to the brain. He is using muscles to walk and hold the radio and eat the candy bar. His hearing, lungs, stomach, and other muscles and glands are functioning simultaneously without any conscious effort.

In a state of hypnosis, all the body and glandular functions can be modified and altered. With the use of hypnosis, the muscles can be made rigid or completely relaxed; pain can be produced or removed; taste can be altered; hearing and speech can be altered, modified, or removed; fear, anxiety, and other emotional problems can be altered or entirely removed; heart rate and breathing can be modified; analgesia and anesthesia can be created; and so with any other symptomatic condition of the human body where a change is desired.

Logic suggests but one conclusion. If all the bodily functions can be altered or changed through the use of hypnosis, then those facilities responsible for the change are also responsible for their continuous functions under ordinary circumstances. The functioning organs, such as the heart, lungs, kidneys, bladder, stomach, and the body in general continue to operate without any conscious effort by the individual. These organs even function during periods of deep sleep or unconsciousness or when one is anesthetized for surgery. The subconscious mind is the energy and impulse directed to the brain, instructing it to perform certain bodily functions by activating the various organs. With the use of proper suggestions made by the subconscious mind while in a state of hypnosis, the function of various organs can be altered or changed.

The function, then, of the subconscious mind is to control the bodily functions, based upon the information as stored in the brain.

The conscious mind is the primary gathering faculty. Whatever a person experiences through the use of his senses, such as sight and hearing, is stored in the brain. Its acceptance is of little consequence in future conduct unless the elements of believability, importance, and truth are included. The conscious mind analyzes the information for believability, importance, and truth. The greater the belief, the greater the future impact on the conduct of the individual. Without the ability to separate the truth from that which is false or the good from that which is bad, chaos would be the result. Most of us have been taught that two plus two is four. However, should someone tell us that three plus three is four and that two plus two is six and those who told us otherwise were lying, we would refuse to accept those statements as being true. Later we would remember the person who made those statements, but it would make little difference because we had refused to accept them as being true.

The subconscious mind also gathers information for storage in the brain's memory bank. However, the difference is that any information the subconscious mind gathers, it does without first analyzing it. The subconscious mind cannot analyze. It either accepts or rejects in total – there is no in-between. The subconscious mind is the secondary gathering faculty,

Consider for a moment that the subconscious and conscious minds are the ends of a balancing scale with the conscious mind as the higher one, and the subconscious mind as the lower one. During normal waking hours, the conscious mind is the primary and predominant one gathering information. This incoming information is analyzed as to believability, importance, and truth. It is accepted or rejected and then stored in the memory bank of the brain. Each one of us on a daily basis performs this function of analyzing incoming information.

Herein lies the difference: What is accepted goes into that part of the memory bank that is intended for future use. When the information is not accepted, this information is automatically rejected into the junk yard, the unimportant section of the brain, not intended for future use. When a person is under stress, anxiety, or other emotional interruption, the analytical portion of the conscious mind is directly affected to the degree that it cannot function efficiently. The greater the stress or emotion, the greater the effect. Under extreme pressure, the conscious mind is almost entirely nonfunctioning. At this point, the conscious mind, having lost its efficiency, begins to lower its side of the scale, causing the subconscious mind to elevate to some point in time during the emotional events; it now becomes the predominant factor. At this point, the conscious mind is in the lower position and the subconscious mind is the primary gathering faculty. Now a person no longer can apply logic to, analyze, or respond to the situation in one's best interest.

We all have been cautioned that if we ever get into trouble, we mustn't panic. The greater the emotional stress, the less logical we become. *It is during these periods of extreme emotional stress that the impressions, impulses, and events become deeply and indelibly imprinted on the memory bank to give rise to future unwanted behavioral responses.* The subconscious mind is neither logical nor analytical. All information, suggestions, or directions that the person is exposed to, are automatically accepted unless the person actively rejects the suggestions or directions.

The primary basis of this rejection is that the suggestions are against self-preservation or against the person's morality. The secondary rejections are when the suggestions are not compatible with the needs and desires of the individual.

With the use of induction techniques, the subject's awareness is transferred from the conscious mind to the subconscious. The directed suggestions of the hypnotist cause the subject to focus his attention in the area dominated by the subconscious mind. Suggestions are made to the subject that his legs are relaxing, arm muscles are relaxing, eyes growing tired, eyelids growing heavy, that his whole body is relaxing and he is going deep, very deep into relaxation. When the subject's eyes close, he shuts out all outside stimuli and focuses his attention on those bodily functions controlled by the subconscious mind. The speed with which the transition is made depends upon the concentration and focus of the subject's attention on his body reaction to the suggestions made by the hypnotist. With his concentrated effort, the subject causes his body to respond to the suggestions of the hypnotist.

By using any one of many induction techniques, the subject voluntarily enters into that state of awareness dominated by the subconscious mind. While he is under stress, the transition is done involuntarily. Whether voluntary or involuntarily, the person is always subjected to the impulses, impressions, and events comprising his surrounding circumstances. Remember, the subconscious mind does not have the capacity to analyze the events taking place and to which the subject is exposed. The truth of the impulse, impressions, or event is not subject to scrutiny and must be rejected or automatically accepted in its entirety. To be rejected, there must be some concerted action taken by the subject. It must be actively rejected. Mere passive rejection is insufficient.

When testing a subject for depth, a suggestion may be made to the effect that the subject is unable to raise his hand or arm, and that the harder he tries, the more difficult it becomes. Should the subject fail to reject this suggestion, the response is usually positive; however, should this subject think he can raise his arm, he will be able to do it. Any and every suggestion addressed to the subject while he is in the state of hypnosis can be rejected depending on the needs and desires for the removal of symptomatic problems. The deeper the state of hypnosis, the more positive the response. It is the conviction of the cure that leads to the cure.

When a person enters the subconscious state of awareness, three things apparently are consistent:
1. There is an increased concentration of the mind.
2. There is an increased relaxation of the entire body.
3. There is an increased susceptibility to suggestion.

The increased concentration is brought about by the elimination of outside stimuli. The person is usually seated in a comfortable chair with the eyes closed. In this situation, there is little or no need for the person's senses to be active. Having the eyes closed shuts out all stimuli, relaxing the optic nerves and all the other thousands of neurons needed for the transmission. The subject's energy can then be concentrated in those areas where it will do the most good.

Concentration and relaxation complement each other. By suggestions, the hypnotist aids the subject in concentrating on relaxing described areas of the body. When each particular area is sufficiently relaxed, then the attention is directed to another area. (In Chapter 11, progressive relaxation is described in detail.) Attention is first directed to eyelids with the suggestion that the subject relax that area. Progressively downward, each muscle and cell are relaxed from the forehead to the toes. By directing the concentration and focusing the attention on each and every area of the body, the subject is relieved of the need to generate thoughts and thereby expend any energy.

The increased susceptibility has caused many serious questions on the acceptability of hypnosis by the general public. The subconscious mind does not have the capacity to analyze the impulses, impressions, or events, and consequently many suggestions, if not rejected, are passively accepted. It is this passive acceptance that has brought about many misconceptions about the use of hypnosis. A person is susceptible to the extent that he desires. Due to the increased need for therapy and removal of symptomatic problems, the subject will not reject almost any suggestion that he believes is necessary in the treatment. The suggestion is further accepted due to the belief and need, and not by any increased gullibility of the person.

A hypnotized person can be dehypnotized at any time he chooses. He can open his eyes and walk about and do anything that he chooses at any time he so elects. Anytime a suggestion or posthypnotic suggestion is given that is contrary to the wishes or beliefs of the subject, it can be voluntarily rejected. If the suggestion is of such a nature that great danger or harm may result, there would be a spontaneous return to the conscious state and the rapport with the hypnotist would be broken by a feeling of mistrust.

Hypnosis is not dangerous; however, careless remarks can lead to psychotherapeutic mismanagement. It is usually the inept therapist or those whose financial benefits are affected who find favor in criticizing hypnosis. All knowledgeable hypnotists agree that when hypnosis is properly administered, according to accepted practices and skill, there is no danger. I personally feel that the danger imputed to hypnosis is an admission of one's inability to obtain satisfactory results. In these cases, the hypnotist is transmitting his own anxieties to the apprehensive subject. No one has ever died from being hypnotized. The same cannot be said about any other form of medicine. There is no modality less dangerous than hypnotism. No therapy is safer.

Hypnosis is, then, a state of awareness dominated by the subconscious mind. All other manifestations in the change of a person's conduct or action are the results of the acceptance of suggestions made during the hypnotic session.

There are several depths of hypnosis, depths of the subconscious mind, just as there are several depths of conscious awareness – that is, perception.

During the conscious state of awareness – that is, when a person is doing his ordinary and normal daily duties – different levels of awareness are experienced. Usually during the morning hours, a person is very active, perceptive, and energetic. As the day progresses, these activities diminish and as the evening hours approach, an individual may become tired and listless to a point where natural sleep is the result. The levels of awareness fluctuate, depending on the importance of the event.

Likewise, there are various levels of awareness that are experienced by the subconscious mind. The longer an individual remains in a state of hypnosis, the deeper he will go and the better the achieved results will be. Experience has proven that the more often one is hypnotized, the faster and deeper the successive sessions will be.

Many attempts have been made to standardize and classify the various levels or depths of hypnosis. Although every writer may have his own classification depending upon his own successes, generally the following classification has been accepted and used as a working basis:

Light: This first level of hypnosis is recognized by the fluttering of the eyelids. Pupils of the eyes recede upward. In this state, most individuals who are apprehensive or not completely ready to accept hypnosis will experience a return to the conscious state. There is an outward appearance of relaxation.

Mild: The relaxation becomes more pronounced, and the breathing appears easier and restful. The arms and legs take on an appearance of complete relaxation, with the possibility of the neck muscles relaxing and a lowering of the head. In testing for this depth, there are the limb and eye catalepsy with a possibility of glove anesthesia. With proper suggestion, the subject will have difficulty in lifting his arms or legs, or opening his eyes.

Medium: With the use of any initial deepening processes as outlined in this book, the following may be successfully obtained: partial amnesia, partial anesthesia, and personality changes. Simple posthypnotic suggestions may also be carried out. In this state, the speech is subdued, and the arms completely and entirely limp.

Deep: Outward physical appearances between this state and the medium state are not easily detected. A relaxation of the facial muscles will appear with the separation of the lips. The face will take on a pale appearance, with most of the flush disappearing. Most of the posthypnotic suggestions will be carried out in detail. Positive and negative hallucinations can be created. This depth must necessarily be obtained to secure the best results in the treatment of psychosomatic disorders. This is the most favorable and accepted state to control smoking and weight problems. Some refer to this state as somnambulism.

Esdaile: This depth of hypnosis is not usually sought or needed for most therapeutic purposes. Most hypnotists are unable to secure this depth in the subjects due to the lack of patience and understanding of the language necessary to obtain its benefits. This state was named after Dr. James Esdaile who performed several hundred major operations on patients with only hypnosis as an anesthetic. It produces exceptional conditions for exceptional purposes.

Success depends on the ability to secure the necessary depth. Failure is the result of attempting to obtain certain responses without first recognizing the depth of the subject. The medium depth is sufficient and adequate for obtaining relaxation of the body and freedom from apprehension and anxiety. Since the procedure to take the subject down to the deepest depth requires only a few minutes, I feel that the excellent results are vital enough and valuable enough to warrant the time expended.

The response of the subject depends upon his own personal characteristics, such as knowledge of hypnosis, fears, misconceptions, and neuroses, as well as his rapport with the hypnotist. Many of these factors vary from day to day in the same person and from subject to subject, producing a variation of responses of the subject from one session to another.

3

Why Hypnosis Works

Nothing should be omitted in an art which interests the whole world, one which may be beneficial to suffering humanity and which does not risk human life or comfort.

— Hippocrates

We have always believed that self-preservation was the first law of conscious existence and that every living conscious creature would express this instinct when faced with life-threatening danger, and would do so without having any special stimulus to bring it into play. There are also other normal and natural instincts common to all human beings which are the products of our present higher form of our evolved existence.

One such universal instinct is to follow or refuse to follow, accept or refuse to accept information without first carefully analyzing this information as to its intent and ultimate purpose. The acceptance of any information will depend on certain underlying factors, such as the status of the person conveying the information, the past education of the recipient, and the importance of the information in the health and happiness of the individual.

Hypnosis has been utilized in one form or another since the beginning of mankind by both medical and religious healers. The one common denominator of these treatments makes full use of the imaginative process to cause the subject to expect a cure. Conviction of cure leads to cure. The subject or patient is not being treated *by* hypnosis but *in* hypnosis. Hypnosis in itself does not cure, but it allows the subject a clearer view of his problems with the ability to meet his needs with new understanding. The new and modern hypnotic techniques are primarily oriented around the needs of the patient rather than being directed by the hypnotist. These factors, together with the use of self-hypnosis, have resulted in a type of hypnotherapy that is completely different from that used by Freud and others.

Critics of hypnosis have been unable to realize that the hypnotic state is a meaningful interpersonal relationship involving real patient participation. Because of the patient's increased receptivity and genuine therapeutic needs, the productive involvement of the patient with the hypnotist results in a ready acceptance of the suggestions.

Each and every person is the architect of his own destiny, and each person has the creative power to make mental images. These mental images are an expansion of the thoughts, needs, and desires to be achieved. By impressing these concepts, needs, and desires upon the subconscious mind, one can cause the visualized condition to be created. Creative energy is the self-induced action of the mind upon itself and within itself. Thought is the power, energy, and force upon the brain, creating all progress and achievement. Nothing in the whole world has ever or will ever be done that is not the result of the mind action known as thought process. The thought comes first, and the action or response follows. Mind power is energy and as energy, it cannot be destroyed.

In the beginning, each of us was only one little fertilized egg. As that cell grew to a certain size, it divided in half, creating two independent cells. Each of these two cells grew to a predetermined size and then again divided in half. And so the process continued until a mature person evolved. Each cell is destined to become a separate and distinct part of the human body. The entire process of growth is a systematic, intelligent pattern of development. This development illustrates the process of life creating life out of itself for a selective purpose. This life-making process of each cell which creates additional cells, is the result of some organized thought and direction. It seems only logical that whatever supervises the present day-to-day functions is responsible for its creation. The heart, lungs, kidneys, liver, bladder, and all the other body organs continue to function daily without any conscious effort. Through the use of hypnosis, the function of each and every organ and gland can be modified. Whatever is responsible for the change is also responsible for its function.

We have but one mind divided into two components: the conscious and the subconscious. Each has the same yet yet different faculties. The conscious mind is that faculty used to gather and analyze information for storage in the brain's memory bank, and the subconscious mind is that faculty that uses the stored information to operate the body process. When the conscious mind becomes impaired or inefficient due to stress, emotion, or drugs, the subconscious mind then receives this information for deposit in the brain's memory bank.

The conscious and subconscious minds function similarly to balancing scales. During ordinary and normal everyday events, the conscious mind is in the dominant position, gathering information, events, impressions, and perspectives. While the absorption of this data is taking place, the analytical power examines this data to determine its believability, importance, and truth. After this analysis is made, the information is then stored in the brain's memory bank for future use, depending upon the relationship of each bit of information to the other information in the scale of importance. In every moment of our conscious awareness, thousands of bits of information are gathered within fractions of a second and as these events continue to unfold, each is analyzed and subsequently stored. The subconscious mind, in turn, then uses this information to regulate body function and emotion. The conscious mind deposits, and the subconscious mind uses. The priority of usage depends upon the relationship of all data in order of believability, importance, and truth.

The conscious mind represents the cognitive activity of our awareness and exercises its powers of reasoning, logic, evaluation, and deduction (just to name a few) objectively before this information is deposited in the memory bank for future use. This conscious mind is the controlling factor that critically evaluates all matter prior to passing on its merits.

Although all information is stored, most of this data is delegated to the junkyard of the memory bank – that is, the area that holds information that is not likely to be used in the future. Basically, the conscious mind refuses to accept any information for future use until it has been determined upon initial entry that this information is believable, important, and true. Information that is deemed to be believable, important and true is deposited in a special place in the memory bank reserved for information to be used in the future.

Each of us determines the relevance of incoming information and its importance to our well-being. The most important factor is believability, and one's belief determines one's behavior. If we consciously recognize information as being believable, important, and true, it impacts our behavior.

In contrast, the subconscious mind functions in an entirely different way. The subconscious mind, or inner mind, serves as a transmitting station from the memory bank to the brain for control and perpetuation of health and well-being. The subconscious mind directs body function, conversion, regeneration, and subjective emotion.

Since the brain rules and controls each and every cell in the whole body, some energy, impulse or direction must be conveyed to the brain authorizing action or inaction. Nothing is automatic. All body responses or emotional conduct is a product of intentional or unintentional direction, conscious or subconscious effort. The subconscious directs the brain into activity by feeding back prior acquired data or commands. These commands may be presently formed or of long standing, only to emerge upon a given time or event. The more believability and importance assigned to this data, the faster the response. So in our normal and everyday activities, the conscious mind is in the dominant position while the subconscious mind occupies that of the subordinate.

When our conscious awareness loses its ability to critically evaluate present activities, a remarkable phenomenon begins to take place within our consciousness.

As our conscious awareness is diminished, the ability to evaluate believability, importance, and truth is substantially affected. The lowering of the conscious awareness automatically elevates the subconscious awareness, working somewhat like balancing scales: when one is lowered, the other rises to the position of dominance. This change depends solely upon the awareness of the conscious mind. The subconscious merely rises or lowers its position depending upon the stimuli directed to the conscious awareness.

This change can be created in only two different and distinctive methods: (1) when the individual is exposed to a traumatic or stressful situation and (2) by design. The greater the stressful situation, the more drastic the change. In any stressful situation, the fight-or-flight syndrome begins to manifest itself. When the individual stands his ground and fights, the conscious mind elects to retain control over the situation or event and refuses to surrender its reasoning or deductive powers. However, when the event is more than the conscious mind can cope with, it begins to retreat and recede within, turning control of body responses and emotional conduct over to the subconscious mind. This is unintentional hypnosis. Children are prone to enter into this state easily and quickly as their deductive and cognitive powers have not been fully developed.

The second method of creating the change is where the conscious awareness is purposely reduced or diminished by suggestions or creative imagery, usually directed by a hypnotist, together with suggestions of relaxation.

When the eyelids are closed, over 240 million cells called rods and cones (sensitive to light, color, and movement) are shut down. In addition, over 30,000 optic nerves that convey messages from the eyes to the visual cortex become inoperative. Closing of the eyelids reduces our conscious awareness by one-eighth. Focusing or concentrating one's attention on a certain area of the body with the intention of creating a feeling of relaxation deprives the other body areas of their reception to outside stimuli. As the outside stimuli are progressively reduced, the individual proceeds into a deeper state of hypnosis.

In this state of relaxation, the subconscious has achieved the position of dominance while the conscious mind has been reduced to the subordinate position previously occupied by the subconscious. At this lower level, the conscious mind no longer possesses the capacity to accumulate information, impulses, or impressions on the cognitive or deductive level. Once attaining the level of dominance, the subconscious mind not only gathers all information but uses this data in forming its commands to the brain to create action or inaction. The subconscious mind at no time ever acquires the capacity to exercise analytical, cognitive, or deductive powers over the newly acquired information. All information is either accepted or rejected in full.

Although all information and events gathered by the conscious mind are deposited in the memory bank for storage, only such information that the conscious mind considers as being believable, important, and true is used by the subconscious mind in creating responses and emotions. Basically, all information is designed to end up in the junkyard of our memory banks except such matters that contain those elements of believability, importance, and truth. These are rescued and saved for future use. The subconscious mind does not possess the same analytical or deductive powers as the conscious mind. So while the conscious mind basically rejects the believability of all incoming information until first it has been scrutinized and analyzed with all previously acquired and stored information, the subconscious, in contrast, accepts everything, rejecting for future use only those suggestions and information that are against the natural law of survival and against the recipient's principles of moral code.

All information, data, or suggestions, whether true or false, once accepted by the subconscious, are deposited in the memory bank as absolute truth. The subconscious mind is further limited in its degree to reject by the depth of hypnosis. The deeper the state of hypnosis, the quicker the acceptance and the faster or more profound the response. A suggestion, for example, that the subject is unable to open the eyelids does result in the subject's inability to do so. Additional suggestions that the harder one tries, the more difficult the task will be, render all attempts futile.

The hypnosis and medical professions have been negligent in failing to recognize the full potential of the state of hypnosis. While we have understood that glandular activity can be inhibited, we have been lax in experimenting with the probable increase of glandular function in hypnosis.

In December of 1986, I traveled to Tucson, Arizona, to treat a young male who had been paralyzed as a result of a surfing accident while visiting a relative in California. This 22-year-old male had sustained a broken neck and some spinal cord damage. For almost three years, he had been confined to a wheelchair, unable to walk. The hypnotic session revealed that following the accident, he was taken to a Los Angeles hospital and during the course of the surgery, the attending physician remarked that the patient would never walk again. The anesthetic administered prior to surgery had rendered the conscious awareness useless, thereby elevating the subconscious mind to the point of dominance. The statement that he would never walk again was accepted by the subconscious mind, and the remark was deposited into the memory bank as an absolute truth. Since the act of walking is a function of the subconscious mind, the only message thereafter conveyed to the brain was the inability to move the muscles necessary to walk. No conscious effort could remove that statement and allow him to walk. During the hypnotic session, he was regressed back to the operating room and revealed the statement of the surgeon, together with other remarks of the severity of the damage. Statements minimizing the nature of the damage were introduced, together with suggestions that such minor injury could not prevent him from continuing to walk normally, that he has restored his body to as good a condition as it was in prior to the accident, and that he is able to stand and walk as he had on several hundred prior occasions without any conscious effort. In less than three hours, he was out of the wheelchair, standing, and with some assistance, was able to move about. He never returned to the wheelchair again.

A wife of a cancer patient of mine called one morning informing me that her husband had not had a bowel movement for three days, even though he had been taking his daily medication. Following a two-hour session at his home, he had a bowel movement and as his wife put it: "It was fifteen inches long, the size of a half dollar, and hard as concrete." He simply sat down and passed it without any effort. He had been reminded on several prior occasions that the nature of his ailment would produce periods of constipation. These suggestions were erased and suggestions given that each and every morning, he does have a bowel movement without any effort as this is a natural and regular function of the body.

At any level of hypnosis, whether induced or accidental, the subconscious mind is open and receptive to the acceptance of any and all suggestions or information without discretion, rejecting only those basically evil and unhealthy, thus following the natural law of survival. As this depth of the hypnotic state increases, the acceptance and responses to suggestions are proportionately affected.

While the conscious mind is not predictable in its direction, varying unexpectedly from one direction to another, the subconscious is definitely very predictable. In some cases, this subconscious level of awareness fits precisely in a pattern. Whatever and whenever the subconscious creates an image of belief, it will cause the conscious mind to transform itself to fit that image or belief. Belief in success tends to produce success. Another one of those predictable patterns of conduct occurs when the subconscious fear produces a fearful behavior. Fear of failure does produce failure. The probably most recognized pattern is that the subconscious refuses to surrender activity or function primarily reserved for the subconscious mind. Walking, for example, is a function of the subconscious, and any attempt to consciously move the muscles in an effort to walk produces an awkward response. The harder one tries, the more difficult the task becomes.

Recently in *Discovery* magazine, there appeared an article describing experiments by scientists. It seems that the subjects of the experiments could recall instructions after having been administered drugs that completely anesthetized them. After the administration of the drugs, they were instructed to rub their ears upon awakening. Upon awakening, nine of the ten subjects performed the instructed task. This, together with other experiments, led the scientists to believe that the conscious mind was not active while in a drugged state. This fact has been known and accepted by hypnotists for many years.

Over twenty years ago, I was called into a hospital to work with a woman whose back had just been operated on for the removal of a cyst. Following the surgery, she was unable to move her legs and was completely paralyzed from the hips down. In hypnosis, she revealed that during the surgery one of the surgeons stated that he hoped she could walk better. However, the patient didn't hear the entire sentence – only hearing that he hoped she could walk. Immediately she believed that something had gone wrong during the surgery and she couldn't walk. Her belief led her to become paralyzed. During the hypnotic session, reason and analyses were injected, thereby removing her misconception of the doctor's remarks. She immediately recovered and in a few days left the hospital.

The subconscious mind, which is responsible for the continuous body function, never rests. When it ceases to function, the person is dead.

The subconscious mind not only hears what has been said, but also knows how you feel about the statement and if you believe what has been said. The conscious part of the mind may misinterpret or misunderstand the message of the subconscious part of the mind, but the reverse is never true.

Through the use of any one of a number of induction techniques, the subject's focus of attention is directed and the outside stimuli limited or removed. When the attention is directed and focused, the subject makes the transition from the conscious awareness to the subconscious awareness. He has entered into a state of hypnosis. As a result of suggestions made by the hypnosis directed to the subject, the latter's critical portion of the conscious mind – that part that does the analyzing – is temporarily suspended and subsequent suggestions are directed to the subconscious mind. Each and every suggestion accepted by the subconscious mind is recorded as true in the brain's memory bank. Having accepted the suggestions, the subconscious mind then directs the brain to create such bodily functions to carry out the terms of the suggestion or suggestions. With the continuous relaxation of the body tissues, through deepening techniques, the subconscious energy is reserved and redirected to carry out therapeutic suggestions.

The conscious mind must operate within a limited power and restriction; however, the subconscious mind knows no such limitations. The power of the subconscious mind is only limited or restricted by the assumption of the conscious mind. Should the conscious mind believe and set limitations on one's endeavors or activities and this belief is placed in the memory bank of the brain, the subconscious mind is limited in potential. However, this limitation may be removed by a direct suggestion to the subconscious mind when in a state of hypnosis. Upon acceptance of the suggestion, all restrictions are immediately removed and set aside, leaving the subconscious free to perform such acts or duties suggested.

The law of success involves just one thing: how you think. You become what you think about. By these thoughts, needs, and desires, the future is created. The future illness or health, wealth or poverty, success or failure depend upon the thoughts and images created, believed, and stored in the memory bank.

The degree of success in hypnosis depends upon each individual's needs, desires, and beliefs. Two things are absolutely necessary: (1) the desire to accomplish something and (2) the belief in what is desired. Without these two elements, the hypnotic session is doomed to failure from its very inception. Hypnosis doesn't work for everyone because everyone doesn't have the desire or belief in what they seek. A person cannot be helped through hypnosis to stop smoking because the spouse doesn't like the smoke or the smell. The desire and belief must be within the person seeking assistance.

The first principle of success is the commitment of the individual, his persistent need, and the desire for something he does not now have. Failure can be overcome by giving the subconscious mind the food for thought, the will to succeed, and the desire to overcome.

Perhaps the greatest and biggest mistake we make is the failure to recognize and understand that the mind has the ability to redirect and recreate itself. Giving the mind adequate and proper recognition and understanding of the nature and function of it will permit you to achieve whatever you desire for growth and enhancement. The function of each and every cell in the human body can be stimulated and affected by the application and addition of drugs and chemicals. Likewise, the function of each cell can be altered, changed, and modified by mental impulses. To direct and sustain the functions of each cell in the human body is beyond the ability of the conscious mind. Research and experiments have led us to believe that the subconscious mind transcends all limitations of space and time.

Recently, following a lecture I gave at a university, I hypnotized one of the instructors. With the use of direct suggestion, I had her visualize and imagine leaving the room and taking a taxicab to the airport and flying to California. Upon arrival in California, she again took a cab to her son's house. She found her son sitting in a chair drinking a can of beer. She further noticed that half of the lawn had been cut, and the lawn mower stood nearby. The clothes that her son wore were described in detail. This woman was then directed to take a cab back to the airport and follow the return route back to the university. Immediately following the session, she was requested to call her son with the instructions that when he answered the phone, she was to ask him to put away the beer and finish cutting the grass. Needless to say, the son was totally amazed that the mother knew of his activities. He wasn't convinced that she was not at his neighbors until he made a return telephone call to her some two thousand miles away. Her description of his activities and dress was flawless. I have performed this experiment hundreds of times and each time continue to amaze the subject. The subconscious mind is not limited to the confines of the skull. Its potential is unlimited.

Suggestions are the key and the solution in problem solving with hypnosis.

The only successful way to impose our thoughts or ideas upon the mind of another is to present those thoughts or ideas in such a subtle manner that they will be accepted willingly by the other with full approval and cooperation before he has time to analyze or reject it. While in a state of hypnosis, the subconscious mind lacks the ability to analyze, and thus it accepts or rejects the suggestion in its entirety. The acceptance of the suggestion urges immediate compliance because the natural function of the subconscious mind is improvement and self-preservation. When a potent and powerful suggestion or idea is suggested, it is more readily accepted and acted upon if the subject believes it is for his betterment and in conformance with his own thoughts and ideas. The closer the suggestion follows the conception of the subject's own logical reasoning, the easier the acceptance and action. Because these thoughts are directed along his own conceived and developed ideas, they are immediately true and in the mind of the subject and worthy of acceptance and compliance. Such an idea, which in fact has no actual or physical basis for its effect, can create a real physiological result. When a thought or suggestion is accepted by the subconscious mind, it is translated into an understanding of its own and it then becomes to that subject an actual living thing according to the interpretation given. The subject's life, health, and social behavior depend not only upon the acceptance of the ideas or suggestions, but also upon his interpretation, understanding, and submission to their natural development.

A prime example of this development is the placebo effect. A person goes to the doctor for examination and treatment of a symptom. Following the examination, the doctor prescribes some medication. When the patient takes the medication, the symptom begins to disappear. The conviction that the medication will cure leads to the cure. The speed with which the symptom will disappear may depend upon the reliability of the physician and the cost of the medication. The medication must be very good if it is expensive.

When a thought, idea, or suggestion is accepted by the subconscious mind, it is automatically and immediately stored in the brain's memory bank to be acted upon by direction. This action may be immediate or delayed, depending upon the need or desire conveyed by the suggestion. This response to the suggestion is an unconditioned behavioral reflex. This reflex can be elaborated and enhanced through the use of deepening processes while in the state of hypnosis. The depth attained has a definite bearing on the results obtained. Hypnosis is a means or artifice used to suppress cortical inhibition and/or rejection and to obtain or achieve a positive response to the behavioral reflex without the interference of the analytical cortex. Spontaneous and unintended occurrences of hypnosis are an indivisible and integral part of our everyday life, resulting in emotional responses and behavioral reflexes in the most intimate events and affections.

It is a fact that most chronic diseases derive their etiology from hypnogenic stimulations either spontaneously induced or provoked. Common manifestations of hypnogenic diseases are anxiety, breathlessness, fatigue, and pain. Each of these symptoms actually occurs in true diseases. Other symptoms may include dizziness, trembling, excessive perspiration or sweating, palpitations, hypertension, and cold or wet hands. Each of these physiological responses could be the result of present-day events associated with events long buried in the memory bank of the same or similar circumstances. In most cases, the hypnogenic diseases are an unintended result.

The placebo effect is the only single action which all drugs have in common and in some cases is the only useful action which the medication can exert. This is the fundamental principle of psychosomatic medicine, administering to the patient an ineffective pill such as a salt tablet in place of an actual drug or medication. It has been well documented that in nogenic situations, which do not require the taking of medications or drugs, the placebo may equally affect the organs and glands of the human body. It is an established fact that body organs and glands respond to impulses arising in the cortex, and these impulses are originally set in motion as a result of the words used by the hypnotists.

Words are the most powerful drugs used by man. There is real magic in the way these words affect the minds of men. We, therefore, as hypnotists, must learn how to use words for the benefit of the subject who is looking forward to some deeply needed assistance. Unfortunately, the hypnotist is usually the last resort instead of the first. Many times I have heard the patient state, "I've tried everything else and if you can't help me, there's nothing left." It then becomes the duty of the hypnotist to choose the words as though he were selecting some prescribed medication, carefully and with precision. Nowhere does the choice of the word mean so much as in hypnosis. Mark Twain once said, "The difference between the right word and the almost right word is like the difference between the lightning and the lightning bug."

Suggestion is nothing more than a group of words assembled to create an idea or image. Suggestion is always with us, but suggestion is very difficult to define. Suggestion may be nothing more than a process of communication resulting in the acceptance with conviction of the idea communicated in the absence of logical reasons for its acceptance.

Since subjects are extremely literal in their interpretation of each and every word made, and because they respond to specific instructions with complete accuracy, words should never be used that may be ambiguous or confusing. Exactness of meaning is essential.

In summary, by means of the induction techniques – that is, the complete focusing of attention and elimination of outside stimuli – the subject gently makes a transition from his conscious awareness to the subconscious awareness, thereby entering into a state of hypnosis. A deepening process is then administered, causing the subject to physically relax and to be mentally removed from the critical faculty of the conscious mind that analyzes words and events. Suggestions are then made in words and phrases readily understandable by the subject. Acceptance of these suggestions by the subject is based upon his needs, desires, and beliefs. Mental images are created in the mind of the subject by the language and suggestions of the hypnotist. The subject then makes his body conform to the subconscious mental image he has of himself. The subconscious mental image then becomes the energy and driving force within, and the end result is that the body emerges as the product of our imagination.

The psychological image causes a physiological change.

4

THE BRAIN

The brain is a collection of nerve cells and can also be defined as simply that part of the nervous system that is contained within the skull. The rest of the nervous system can be found in the spinal cord. Just as our body is divided into two sections, the right and the left sides, so too our brain is divided in half with each side looking almost identical. Without going into great detail, it is important that the hypnotist be aware of the different sections of the brain and their specific functions.

A drawing is provided on the next page to assist in understanding the various sections of the brain and their respective locations.

The Frontal Lobe: This is everything in front of the nervous Sylvian fissure. This area primarily controls the physical movements of the body. In this area, the more complex motor movements are organized, and destruction of any part of this area can lead to partial or total paralysis, depending upon the severity of the damage. In the most forward portion of the frontal lobe, there are prefrontal fibers which exert an inhibitory control over our activities, and any physical damage to this area can cause the individual to act without inhibitions, which results in conduct not in accord with previously controlled responses. The hypnotist's therapeutic suggestions for removal or modification of undesirable inhibitions are directed to this area. Frigid women, fearful of sexual acts caused by previously traumatic experiences, can have their behavioral patterns modified or changed while in a state of hypnosis by not rejecting the proper suggestions that remove any or all inhibitions.

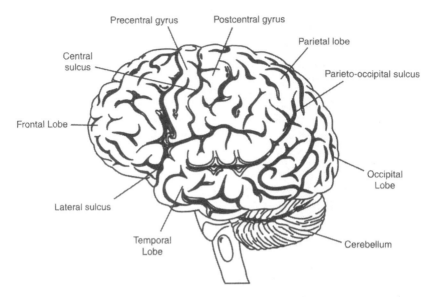

Figure 1. External Anatomy of the Brain

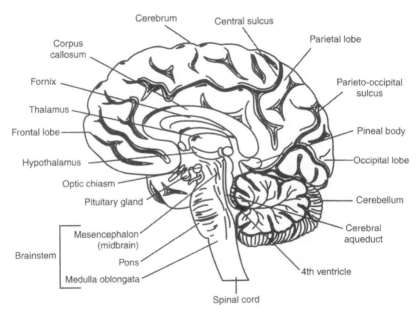

Figure 2. Sagittal Section Through the Brain

The Parietal Lobe: This is the cortical area that lies directly behind the central fissure and contains the primary sensory functions of the brain. This area is very precise in its arrangement as it receives all of the pulses from each and every sensory receptor. This function permits the brain to precisely pinpoint which area of the body is transmitting the sensory impulses. When this area is not intact or is damaged, confusion may result in receiving a message that the toe is injured when, in reality, it is the knee that is affected. Suggestions of analgesia and anesthesia, when properly given, inhibit the function of these sensory receptors and prevent the messages from the affected area being recorded in the brain. A general anesthesia has a similar function by shutting down the message from the area of the surgical procedure to the brain.

The Occipital Lobe: This area is the visual center where the images or signals, conveyed from the eyes by means of the optic nerves, cause incredible transformations and reassembly of the images in the occipital lobe. Damage to this area can or may result in blindness. Hallucinatory suggestions to the subject, while he is in a state of hypnosis, affect the transformation of these images so that they are not reassembled with precision, leading to false impulses. The hallucinatory suggestions are false descriptions, which are accepted by the subject in a state of hypnosis, when the subconscious mind is the dominating faculty. Since the subconscious mind cannot rationalize or analyze, these projected false descriptions, not having been rejected, are accepted as true. Once the mind accepts the suggestions, the images are recorded as true in the occipital lobe.

The Temporal Lobe: This is the area below the Sylvian fissure and involves hearing, memory, time, and individuality. The temporal lobe is a very intriguing part of the brain largely due to its connection with the underlying areas. Its connection with the limbic system permits one to experience anger, hate, fear, and other forms of disturbing emotions. Corrective suggestions in hypnosis are easily accepted by this area, leading to a more productive and enjoyable life.

The Medulla: The medulla is the connecting link between the spinal cord and the brain stem, and at this junction there is an expansion to approximately one inch in diameter. It is through the medulla that all nerve fibers from the two cerebral hemispheres crisscross on the way down to the spinal cord and end up controlling the opposite sides of the body. The duty of the expanded vital flesh, the medulla, is to control functions such as swallowing, talking, breathing, vomiting, and singing. In addition, this area controls blood pressure, respiration, and in some instances the rate of heartbeat. Damage to the area of medulla and brain stem can result in a drop in blood pressure and inability to breathe. When the damage is extensive, death may result in a matter of minutes.

Persons in a terminal state are unable to swallow, resulting in a gradual loss of weight, although there may be nothing physically wrong with the area of the medulla. I have treated terminally ill patients unable to swallow any solid food for months by suggestions to them, while they are in a state of hypnosis, that they were physically capable of swallowing food as they had done more than a thousand times before. For reasons unknown to them, they acquired the belief that they could not swallow and when that belief was buried deep into the brain's memory bank by the repetition of the suggestion, all muscular action in the process of swallowing ceased. Creating a reversal response is a simple procedure. While the patient is in a state of deep hypnosis, the suggestion is made to him that he has the capacity to control various physical movements, even though he is suffering from some ailment, as he has performed the task of swallowing thousands of times before. Swallowing is now just as automatic in nature as moving the fingers, lifting the eyelids, walking, talking, or any other such activity. This suggestion then overshadows the deep-seated belief and restores the normal and natural function of swallowing. As the patient recognizes that he now does have and always had the ability to swallow solid food, the appetite increases and weight is restored. It was the thought and belief that he couldn't swallow that created the initial problem, and the subsequent thoughts removed his impediment. Remember that the changes are made while a person is in hypnosis and not by hypnosis. The medulla is particularly affected by the administration of such drugs as morphine and nicotine. These functional changes are easily recognized in persons who smoke cigarettes and retain an excessive amount of nicotine.

Thalamus: Moving up from the medulla through the brain stem, we reach the thalamus, which is a Greek term meaning "couch." It is in this area that the cerebral hemispheres lie and rest in a comfortable position. All information, except smell, must pass through the thalamus on the way to the cerebral hemispheres for processing.

Hypothalamus: This is the area immediately below the thalamus and is the central control regulator for water balance, endocrine levels, sexual activities, food intake, and the automatic nervous system. In addition, the hypothalamus controls and regulates emotional states such as eating drives, hate, and complacency (just to name a few). The hypothalamus controls and regulates physical activities that accompany emotional states. A nervous person exhibits a fidgety appearance, while a person who has just completed a satisfying meal is relaxed and content. Physical activity is an objective clue of the emotional state of the individual, and an observance of this activity will generally reveal to the hypnotist the basic cause of such conduct. The thalamus and hypothalamus are the most important of all organs to be considered in the use of hypnosis, for the hypothalamus is the center and somewhat controlling factor in these complex, motivational, emotional states.

The spinal cord, which resembles a rope of many fibers, gathers impulses and impressions from the skin and muscles and, in return, sends out messages for physical movement. The brain stem, being a spinal cord, performs similar functions relating to the activities of the head and neck. Other than the senses of vision and smell, the brain stem is the center of all our other senses. The basal ganglia and the cerebellum, working in conjunction with it, coordinate and regulate physical movement.

That by no means concludes all of the various parts of the brain; however, it is sufficient that the hypnotist be aware of the functions and principal areas of the human brain, for it is of such a complex structure that no one will ever possibly grasp its entire nature. We must realize that all of these various parts are joined together to form one continuous system that we call the central nervous system.

The functional arrangement of the nervous system is something like this: The spinal cord and the brain stem, which is the uppermost part of the spinal cord, receive impulses and impressions from the skin and muscles and, in turn, send out requests for physical movement. In addition, the brain stem is the recipient of the information gathered by our senses, except smell and vision which are directly connected to the limbic system and cerebral cortex. All this information is assembled in the thalamus and hypothalamus, and forwarded to the various parts of the brain that control the functions of the body. In addition, the hypothalamus contains other control areas relating to such functions as heart rate, body temperature, and respiration.

It must now be evident that the conduct of the entire nervous system and its related functions are the result of organization and intelligence. Whatever is responsible for the modification must also control the original function. A patient in a state of hypnosis can experience changes in body temperature not consistent with the environment. Two individuals seated in the same room can feel different room temperatures. Heart rate can be modified by suggestion. Positive and negative hallucinations can be experienced. Any and all physical muscular movement can be altered and modified. With the proper use of suggestions, smell and taste can be extremely modified so the individual experiences something entirely different. After having observed the changes in several thousand individuals while in a state of hypnosis, I can only conclude that the subconscious mind is the controller of the functions of our bodies.

The human brain is a cluster of at least ten billion nerve cells called neurons, and each neuron consists of a nucleus, a long fiber (the axon), and an extensive number of dendrites (hairlike extensions) that extend out to contact other nerve cells. Each of the billions of neurons has thousands of connecting points between cells that are called synapses. The total number of synapses in a human brain is almost beyond calculation. There may be as many as 100 trillion synapses in the human brain, receiving and calculating signals arriving as electrical impulses or impressions. When a sufficient number of impulses or signals touch the first neuron, a chemical called a neurotransmitter is released in the form of vesicles. At a particular assigned time, the vesicle releases its packet of transmitters permitting them to transfer to the second neuron. Each transmitter crosses over to its own receptor and by this process will move from one neuron to another until the journey is complete. Some transmitters may be inhibitory in nature which, in turn, shuts down the movement of the original impulse so that the message conveyed to the brain is not received. When a sufficient number of messages are inhibited from progressing, the brain's capacity to process the message is impaired. The rate at which these neurotransmitters travel depends upon the need for physical responses, thus regulating physical movement with the thought process, as both are in harmony with each other.

Injections of chemicals can inhibit or enhance the transmission of neurotransmitters from cell to cell. Hypnosis has a similar effect, depending on the nature of the suggestions and depth of hypnosis. Whatever the chemicals are able to do within the human body, hypnosis can do without side effects.

The brain is an organ developed from a single cell, the egg, and then into a hundred billion cells by means of multiplication. During the nine-month period before birth, the development of the brain accelerates at an incredible rate of 250,000 cells per minute. In the earliest stages, these embryonic cells are free to become components of muscle, skin, or other parts of the body and if such cells are removed and transposed to another part of the body, they would "rethink" themselves and transform into cells appropriate to that area. However, nerve calls can only grow as nerve cells, no matter where they find themselves. Neurons in the brain migrate to other parts of the brain destined to become motor cells, sensory cells, and uncommitted cells. These uncommitted cells serve as connecting cells.

Vision: Vision is the function of the eyes in assembling the various components of the environment surrounding the individual. Light, distance, color, and movements (just to name a few) are gathered and transported by means of the optic nerves to that area in the rear of the brain known as the striate cortex, where the component parts are reassembled to form a picture. This reassembled picture is forever changing as the things observed continue to create a different image. Although everything observed is reassembled and recorded in the brain, only these observations that create stimulation within the sense are acknowledged by the conscious mind. All others are recorded in the brain's memory bank by the subconscious mind. Pictures of delicious food can stimulate the appetite and taste buds. In addition, as we see an object, we can interpret the object's weight. We do so by an analytical process combining the incoming information to arrive at a conclusion. A subject while in a state of hypnosis, having received certain descriptive information, creates a picture or image reflected by his subconscious mind. That image overshadows the true image when the eyes have been opened, resulting in positive or negative hallucinations. The true image or picture is not reassembled due to the interruptions of the transmission. In cases where there is unintentional hypnosis created by fear or anxiety, the visual observations, although properly reassembled and present in the memory bank, prevent a conscious recall of these events. Returning to the state of hypnosis will permit the individual to recall and remember events not heretofore acknowledged in the conscious state.

Movement: Initially, all physical muscular movement has a certain amount of mystery and intrigue. Once one has made the decision, the physical movement begins and the speed of the action depends upon the urgency of the act. After watching television for several hours, there may be some reluctance to get up to do some chores. However, consider the same circumstances upon hearing a window break; there is an instant physical movement of arising. In both instances, there was the initial decision to get up; however, the muscular movement was without any conscious effort as to how the activity was to be carried out. When a person attempts to consciously control muscular movements that are the responsibility of the subconscious, the movements are awkward and clumsy. There is no part of the brain assigned to the decision-making process; however, each component of the brain is controlled by this process. The brain is well organized and complex in the structure, and each level or component of the brain is related in a degree of mutual influence.

Consider for a moment the activity involved in picking up a pencil. First, we observe the pencil and calculate the distance and movement necessary to grasp the object, and then the muscular activity to lift it. In a fraction of a second, a decision is made as to what effort is required. While the initial effort is in progress, follow-up decisions are made on an ongoing basis as the relationship to the pencil changes. Since no conscious effort is extended, what then causes this well-organized movement to be so precise?

Before attempting to arrive at a conclusion, we must realize that in addition to the described movements, there are voluntary and involuntary activities simultaneously being processed by the brain and proceeding independently of each other. Without proper instructions, this activity would end in confusion and disruptive movement. A person in a state of hypnosis is always aware of the circumstances surrounding his activities and that of the hypnotist, yet with proper instructions, his movements can be altered or completely inhibited. These instructions are directed to the subconscious mind and inhibit the activities, even though there are conscious attempts on the part of the subject to perform differently. The conclusion that can be drawn is that the subconscious mind is responsible for these precise muscular movements.

It is interesting to recognize that most of our conscious activities involve many involuntary components, and we are better off performing these activities without the involvement of our consciousness.

The success of simple and complex events depends largely on the precise coordination and movement of the motor, visual, and sensory components of the human body. The needs, desires, images, and beliefs are combined with the physical involvement on a repetitious basis, instilling into the memory bank a pattern of movement that controls similar future activities. A basketball player, for example, simultaneously jumps, turns, lofts, and deposits the basketball into the hoop without any apparent conscious concern; for these reflexes appear to be one continuous, coordinated movement. This remarkable accomplishment is largely due to the cerebellum, an organ which is part of the human brain. The cerebellum is a control center, coordinating the sensory information from every part of the body with the need for motor responses based on the desires and beliefs contained in the memory bank. As this data is gathered in the cerebellum, it is instantly assembled and programmed into signals for muscular movements resulting in an automatic execution of physical activity. Upon forming the intent to perform a movement, coupled with the belief that it can be done, the cortex is activated. These impulses are then sent to the cerebellum through the thalamus. When the coordinated messages are ultimately received by means of impulses, there is muscular activity. One of the miracles of the brain is how it is able to coordinate the activities of vision and movement.

The brain is the most powerful human organ, and yet it is very fickle in the manner that it is affected by the internal and external environment. Light, darkness, time of day, rain, and warmth (just to name a few variables) affect the manner and efficiency of the brain. However, these alone do not influence or control its operation. It is the association of other factors, along with the data stored in the memory bank, that makes up a formula by which the brain must function.

Since the brain controls every cell in the entire human body, it becomes clear to the hypnotist that the more precise the instruction given, the more effect upon each cell. The cells respond in conjunction with the instructions from the brain, and the brain receives its impulses from the subconscious mind. These impulses are the direct result of the combination of the data stored in the memory bank, new impulses or information, and the credibility of the individual data.

When there is a malfunction in the relay of the information from the sensors to the brain and then the brain sends its instruction for action, devastating results may occur. Likewise, when the brain's own cells are malfunctioning due to the process of chemicals taken voluntarily or involuntarily, the physical movements are unpredictable. Any interruption of normal relay of information to the brain and its return to the area of action will cause a variance on the body responses. These interruptions are the result of two separate and distinct causes. The first occurs when there has been a decrease in or damage to the cells in the chain of transmissions. The second occurs where the instruction from the subconscious mind creates a misdirection. *The greatest effect on the human activity is the second. In the absence of cell damage, every act, conduct or activity, whether or not consciously intended, is the direct response from the subconscious mind.*

Pathologists and neuroscientists, after having conducted experiments over the past century on several thousand brains, have concluded that the hypothalamus exerts an ever-increasing influence on the function of the organs of the human body. This tiny organ, only one three-hundredth of the brain, is involved in an enormous number of body activities. The hypothalamus plays an important part in the digestive system, appetite, body weight, ulcers, blood pressure, pulse, temperature, and sexuality (just to name a few). A slight accidental injury or the mere touching of the hypothalamus by a surgeon during a surgical procedure may cause the patient to immediately slip into a coma from which he may never emerge. In addition, the hypothalamus exerts functional control over the pituitary glands. When the blood supply from the hypothalamus to the pituitary is altered, there is a corresponding effect on the function of the pituitary. Since the pituitary glands function in a rhythmic fashion, any disruption of this rhythm prevents normal function and adversely affects sexuality in men and women.

Without going into further detail as to the workings of the hypothalamus, it is sufficient for the hypnotist to understand that there are organs within the human body and especially the brain that control, influence, and regulate other body organs and functions. The hypothalamus may be considered the regulator of these symptomatic functions while the entire brain is somewhat of a mediator.

The limbic system and the frontal lobes are generally associated with our emotions, and when the frontal lobes are damaged or destroyed, the emotions controlled by the frontal limbic connections become unpredictable. This damage to the frontal lobes can bring about chemical imbalance, and any minute change in the chemical or electrical state of the brain results in changes in behavior.

Hypnotists have long recognized that suggestive therapy can lead to instant changes in emotional patterns. I received a call one evening from an individual who was so besieged with guilt, he was on the verge of committing suicide. I had never met this gentleman prior to this evening and upon arriving at his home, I found him to be in a highly emotional state and irrational. I proceeded to hypnotize him and, after a two-hour session, he was calm and stable. The suggested therapy was taped, and he was requested to listen to the tape several times that evening. The next afternoon a second session was conducted and at the conclusion of this session, the individual was calm, logical, and rational. He openly discussed the circumstances leading to his guilt feeling and his suicidal behavior. Logic and reason prevailed, and he now enjoys a productive life. Since the frontal lobes together exert their influence on the hypothalamus, can it be said that in this case, the hypothalamus refused their influence due to the superior influence of the subconscious mind? Emotion is something intangible. It is not material, has no essence, and occupies no space. The mind is also intangible. But the mind, being supreme, creates the emotion in its own image.

Pain is the universal form of stress, and it is a blessing that we are able to recognize this form of stress; for pain is the method of communicating from one area of the body notifying the brain that there is some damage or injury. Without the symptomatic feeling of pain, serious injury could be incurred without recognizing the need for medical attention.

The question may be asked that, once recognizing the injury through the body communication of pain, why must we continue to receive the message? The answer is very simple. We don't have to suffer any continuous pain. The problem lies in one's ability to cancel out the message after the first transmission. Pain in small quantities can be beneficial; however, when taken to extremes, pain can be immobilizing.

The initial step in experiencing pain begins in the complex network of nerve endings distributed throughout the surface of the skin. Rapid conducting fibers carry the message of pain at varying speeds from the surface to the spinal cord for instant transmission toward the brain with termination in the thalamus. The greater part of the brain is not involved and has nothing to do with pain perception. The brain contains and supplies its own opiates, chemical substances that occupy these pain receptors, and prevents the continuous transmission of the message of pain. Narcotics such as morphine or heroin, when administered to the body, occupy additional receptors, and when sufficient receptors are occupied, no further transmission of the message occurs. However, when these opiates are dissipated or when the administered drugs are eventually flushed out of the receptors and organs, then the pain is restored. The administration of the drugs reduces the production of the natural opiates by the brain, leaving the individual more dependent upon the drugs. The pain relief of drugs inevitably is associated with the tendency to take more pain relievers, increasing the dependency factor. Eventually the situation exists where the brain's receptors become totally dependent upon the drugs and when these narcotics become unavailable, the body undergoes nagging withdrawal symptoms.

How is it then possible for hypnosis to play an integral part in relieving the individual from these stress-creating withdrawal symptoms?

Consider for a moment that a person just learned that another with whom he had been intimate was being treated for a sexually transmitted disease such as herpes or AIDS. The very *thought* of the possibility of contracting such a disease instantly, without conscious effort, accelerates the heartbeat as a physical manifestation of the inner feeling of distress. The increase of the heartbeat, or the decrease depending upon the nature of the stress, is affected by the chemicals contained within the heart muscles. The release of these chemicals either stimulates or retards the heartbeat, directly affecting the nervous system and culminating in the discharge of stress-related neurochemicals. This domino effect continues throughout the entire nervous system. Adrenaline is secreted from the adrenal glands into the bloodstream, activating and affecting other glands. Situations or events that are very stressful are associated with an increased risk of other known conditions such as cancer, heart attacks, and a weakened immune system. To state it very simply, harboring and entertaining certain thoughts create a stressful situation, resulting in unnecessary and uncontrolled physical responses. *It is the psychological images that create the physical responses.*

To answer the question of how hypnosis can reduce this domino effect becomes self-evident. Since the body responses follow the thought process, a change in thoughts or ideas will automatically change the body response. Hypnosis utilizes the subconscious mind to deposit a thought into the memory bank of the brain for future use under certain conditions and events. When future responses are predicted, they are referred to as controlled responses. "Attitudes" and "states of mind" can either increase or decrease a person's ability to resist or fight infection or such a devastating disease as cancer.

When a person becomes involved in too many events that are beyond his control, there is a tendency to develop stress-related ailments; for we react to these events instead of treating them in a logical and analytical manner. When a person is exposed to traumatic or frightful events, messages are passed through the nervous system from the brain, producing adrenaline which, in turn, increases the heartbeat. The adrenal glands are further stimulated, giving off adrenaline which is discharged into the bloodstream and maintains the rapid heartbeat to induce physical responses such as trembling and sweating. Drugs known as beta blockers may be administered to prevent the adrenaline from reaching its receptors and causing the heartbeat to speed up. However, the prevention of the normal interrelationship of the adrenaline and the noradrenalin by the administration of the beta blockers can have serious and harmful effects on the body as a whole.

The heartbeat of an individual can be increased or decreased by suggestion alone while in a state of hypnosis. Accepted suggestions of relaxation and comfort are all that is necessary to create a calm and pleasant feeling upon the happening of an event. Speaking before a group for most persons creates tension, apprehension, and anxiety. These feelings can be reduced and, in some cases, entirely removed with the use of proper suggestive therapy while the patient is in a state of hypnosis. The thoughts and images deposited in the memory bank control the future responses at the happening of the event. Having undergone suggestive therapy, the same person, relaxed and confident, gives his lecture before an audience. The fearful thoughts are no longer present to cause the production of noradrenalin or adrenaline.

Concentration plays an ever-increasing role in the performance of an athlete. Concentration is the thought process by which the outside stimuli are removed or reduced and when concentration is uninterrupted, the performance is graceful and successful. However, when concentration is broken, attention is shifted, allowing thoughts of failure and doubt to enter, which result in lost confidence and control. Without concentration, confidence, and control, the physical ability is impaired, leaving the person in a panic situation. Hypnosis permits the person to enter a state of rest and relaxation, removes the feeling of panic and failure, and restores confidence and control. Hypnosis modifies the brain's reaction to stress by establishing a relaxation response. Unfortunately, persons suffering from stress and its related symptoms turn to drugs and other chemicals for relief instead of their own abilities to offset the impact of these stressful events. Each of us has the capabilities to control our bodily emotions and responses, and the time should be taken to learn how to put this powerful tool to work.

Each living moment, the brain is bombarded with thousands of new facts, impulses, impressions, ideas, and events for storage and future use. A computer has recently been developed that can process billions of calculations per minute, and this hardly touches the potential of the brain. The conscious mind, that part of our awareness primarily responsible for gathering information, instantly computes incoming information with the prior stored data for credibility and effect. This information is categorized and stored in the memory bank for future use. Considering the speed with which this information is gathered and analyzed, one can understand that at times, we are not conscious of all that has been assembled for storage in the memory bank. Usually one single bit of information is recollected and, based upon that one piece, another fact is added until the whole picture is recreated. The recalling of a single fact, image, or impression which was originally deposited in the memory bank through the sensory facilities may bring about the recollection of other similar events long ago. Although the recollection of a single fact may not necessarily recreate the entire picture, one does get the feeling that there is some relationship between the current and the distant events without recognizing the relationship.

During an interview, a patient expressed some concern about her growing dislike for her minister, whom she only met during church services. She was hypnotized and age-regressed in search of some initial sensitizing event not related to this dislike. Upon her reaching the eighth grade, the problems of her schooling were discussed, and she started to sob and cry. She had a distinct recollection of her stepfather waving his arms, shouting, and criticizing her unnecessarily. Before she started the ninth grade, her stepfather left, never to be seen again. The minister's use of certain words and his waving of the arms reminded the subconscious mind of her stepfather and recreated the feeling of intense dislike within the patient. This dislike was transferred to the minister without any conscious awareness.

Another patient was brought in to see me by her children who expressed some concern about her mental stability. They explained that she was shopping for some pictures to hang on the wall when suddenly she screamed and ran out of the store. Subsequent questioning failed to reveal any clues to explain her conduct. She was regressed to age thirteen when she explained that there was an attempted molestation and from her position on the couch, she saw a picture on the wall just above her. She had observed the identical picture in the department store. Looking up at this picture brought forth deep emotional memories, causing her to react in the same manner as she did during the molestation.

Memory is stored and locked within the brain, and the emotions and moods existing at that time accompany this data into the storage bank. Some of these memories are so wrapped up in emotion and there is an attempt to bury the events so deeply, they cannot surface at some future date. Patients suffering from depression, anxiety, and tension do so because several such events have been accumulated within the memory bank and, when coupled with the emotions, an uncontrolled reaction is set in motion. These eventful emotions were buried without the benefit of logic and reason, and resulted in uncontrolled reactions. While a person is in a state of hypnosis, the mere recalling of a traumatic event is not in itself sufficient to remove the accompanying emotions. Logic and reason must be inserted into this memory recall to remove reactions and restore control within the patient. In the previous example, logic and reason would state that the stepfather is long gone and she is no longer a child but a mature adult who must be able to assert her position; and if the need arises, assistance can be obtained. All the memory recall of shouting and waving of the arms can do her no harm. She is free to do the things she desires without fear of condemnation. How can the picture on the wall cause harm? Neither the picture nor the couch nor any other item within the picture of the initial event can now hurt her. She has been removed from that event. Neither the past nor the future but only the present must be addressed and considered. Logic is inserted into the thoughts by making logical statements. Reasoning is explaining the present conditions and how they vary from the past and that the past should have no effect on today's events.

While one is in a hypnotic state, the intensity of the painful past experiences can be modified and reduced in intensity, relieving the patient from recurring emotions when associated events are recognized.

Of all our senses, sight is the most likely to be associated with memory recall; for we tend to remember those events that are most important and that have created an image concept. Memory recall is the reconstruction of original images and the more often the picture is recreated, the more detailed it becomes. *Repetition, while in a state of hypnosis of the therapeutic suggestions, creates an immediate and constant controlled response at some future event. Self-hypnosis is the means of assuring that these responses be maintained continuously.*

Memory recall and the retention of new information depend largely on the condition of the brain. We refer to the brain as the overall body of the organ, but the brain is divided into several subsystems, each having its own particular and peculiar function in the memory process. Damage, injury, or disease in one area of the brain may affect only a portion of the memory and recall operation; however, when this does occur, the memory function may be carried out by another area somewhat distant from the affected portion. The left and the right portions of the brain have this tendency to compensate for each other in the event of damage or injury to the corresponding area on the opposite side.

Every memory stimulus, regardless of its origin, takes a more or less circuitous route by which it finally reaches its storage bank. Those stimuli, such as smell and taste, that take the shorter route have a more distinct character for recall. If emotion is involved during the event, the probability of recall is greater. Unfortunately, the ability to recall also revives those emotional responses to a certain degree. The desire to "bury" or "forget" events that are associated with extreme emotional responses varies with the extent or degree of the symptom. Nothing is "forgotten." It is our accessibility to the memory that is impeded.

Memory is the thought process that controls and regulates our behavior, our performance, our personalities and every act, whether it is simple or complicated. These patterns of behavior become established as the brain records the experiences and knowledge gathered over the life of the individual. These patterns of behavior then become "programs of conduct" that precisely control future conduct. Should the patient or subject desire a change in conduct, then it becomes the hypnotist's duty, using hypnotherapy, to change programs of conduct.

Although neuroscientists have determined that the two hemispheres of the brain, the left and right, are responsible for separate and distinct functions, they are in agreement that we need both sides, as the hemispheres tend to complement each other in this vast network of transmitters and receptors. What remains unsolved is the purpose of this crisscross pattern of interacting nerve fibers from the spinal cord up and into the brain. Hypnotists deal only with the function of this network of nerve fibers and not with its structural nature.

Many hypnotists, physicians, and others consider hypnosis a state of altered consciousness; however, I must take issue with this interpretation. The administration of drugs, including alcohol, alters our conscious awareness and causes changes in our brain wave patterns, resulting in the disappearance of the normal alpha rhythm and registering the appearance of the lower beta activity. Every alteration or change in awareness is not accompanied by a change in the brain's electrical activity. Hypnotized persons, for example, do not register such changes but continue to show a normal brain wave pattern.

Neuroscientists have been unable to determine why some changes in awareness produce alterations in brain activity while others have no effect. The answer has always been present, but it has eluded them, for they fail to recognize anything but organic activity. Many scientists believe that nothing exists other than the brain's reaction to some external or internal reality. The brain is responsible for all behavioral patterns, for that is the basic purpose of the brain's existence. The mind is the creator of the thought process, the energy source that directs and instructs the brain to perform certain functions at any given time. The subconscious mind directs the so-called "automatic" functions, while the conscious mind controls the decision-making process. Whenever a decision is made and transferred to the subconscious mind by acceptance, the resulting physical response becomes automatic. Thoughts create brain activity and, without a thought, brain activity is impossible. Although the subconscious and the conscious minds function independently, they are always in harmony in brain activity. A conscious decision is made to reach down to the floor and pick up something. Instantly and almost concurrently, the physical movement commences, activating certain muscles to carry out this desire. *Such physical movement of the muscles is without conscious effort; the only conscious activity is the creation of the intent.*

A person in an unconscious state has lost the use of his conscious mind or conscious awareness. The subconscious mind continues to function in all states except death. A patient undergoing a major surgical procedure, totally anesthetized and in an unconscious state, records and stores in the brain's memory bank all activity within the operating room. The subconscious mind is always and ever alert to the impulses and impressions within the senses' receptors.

I had a visit from a patient, involved in an automobile accident, who had a desire to recall the events leading up to the accident. He had no recollection of the accident and the four days following his collision. In hypnosis, he remembered every bar he had visited and each person with whom he had any contact. He was able to recall all of the events leading up to the accident and in addition, he remembered the paramedics treating him and his ride to the hospital. His state of awareness had been so inhibited by the alcohol he had consumed that he was not consciously aware of any of these events. His subconscious mind was open, alert, and receptive to all of the incoming impulses and recorded them without any conscious awareness.

The brain is a powerful and complex organ with capabilities beyond our imagination. These capabilities are limited by the belief that certain acts or functions cannot be performed. Change the belief and we change the result.

References

Restak, Richard M. *The Brain: The Last Frontier*. New York: Doubleday & Co., 1979.
Restak, Richard. *The Brain*. New York: Bantam Books, 1985.
Rose, Steven. *The Conscious Brain*. New York: Alfred Knopf, 1973.
Yates, Francis A. *The Art of Memory*. Boston: Routledge and Kegan Paul, 1966.

5

STRESS—OVERREACTIVITY

All disease has a component of overreactivity or stress at the very cause.

Researchers now – and have for some period of time – concentrated their attention on the cause of the disease rather than the diseased cells or the symptoms. We have long recognized that each of us has an immune and defensive system consisting of billions of cells that form the army within to protect the individual from invaders and to heal any damaged areas. The function of the immune system is to rid the body of foreign and injurious material such as a virus, germs, bacteria, and the like. This has become more and more evident with the transplant of human organs. Recognizing that these transplants are not of the body tissue, a great deal of effort is exerted on the part of the immune system to reject these organs and make them become nonfunctional. In order to offset this rejection, certain medication is administered to retard the workings of the immune system in order for the transplanted organ to gain some credibility within the body's process. However, by diminishing the effect of the immune system, the rest of the body becomes easy prey for any and all other diseases or malfunctions. This, in turn, requires constant monitoring of the body function to maintain an even balance between the immune system and the donated organ.

Recognizing that not only drugs can affect the functioning of the immune system, researchers in medicine have determined that stress and overreactivity equally have an enormous effect on this defense system of the body. This stress and overreactivity has a domino effect. In other words, a chain reaction is set in motion that allows for a progressive deterioration or additional stress by being stressful in the first place.

Stress, exhaustion, overreaction, and *burnout* are terms most commonly associated with the physical condition where the body is not functioning at its most efficient capacity. What creates the degree of stress, frustration, or overreaction for us besides our own home life, personal, or social lives, or work situation is pretty much uniform to any human being. Over the years, either through publicity or our own personal experiences, we recognize certain jobs or job-related situations as being more stressful than others. Air traffic controllers, firefighters, police officers, and emergency rescue teams fall within that category because of particular events with which we can identify them or that we become aware of with regard to their responsible obligations.

No situation in itself need be stressful. The main problem is that we as individuals do not know how to handle the situation or our reactions associated with a particular situation which, in turn, leads us to conclude that this situation is stressful and we have no control over it. When we accept this, then all such situations can create overreaction and stress, and we become aware of our stressful reaction. Once having become aware of our reaction, we tend to seek help to relieve ourselves of this unnecessary symptom of anxiety and stress. Help may be in the form of a doctor, a vacation, alcohol or other drugs, a change of environment. If the condition is not severe, then a vacation may be sufficient to rejuvenate the body. The use of drugs, including alcohol, merely tends to delay the inevitable need for some form of relief. The symptoms are inhibited, but the problem or the cause of the stress and overreaction still remains. Using drugs allows one to keep going, even though his system is still continuing to overreact. The action or overreaction of individuals in relation to the information stored in their memory bank may be divided into two different and distinct categories.

The two major problems of society today are mental and physical. Stress and overreaction, however, are a combination of these two: mental first and then physical. Generally these categories are split, but there is some overlapping. People generally have a tendency to think their attitude, their reaction, and their feelings about stress and overreaction are largely dictated by however they categorize it.

Should the problem of stress and overreaction be considered by the individual to be physical, then a physician is generally consulted. After the doctor has run tests, secured X-rays, and conducted a physical examination, he is expected to reach a diagnosis. Once the diagnosis has been ascertained, a cure is expected. The cure is usually in the form of medication. We expect to put our problems in the hands of the doctor who is supposedly trained to cure our ailments. In other words, we expect the doctor to handle the situation.

Once there has been a determination that the problem of stress or overreaction is physical, two reactions occur. The first is that the individual can't do anything about it, and the second is that the doctor will handle the problem. In effect, we have over the years placed in our brain's memory a suggestion that is now controlling our future conduct, once we have determined that the condition from which we are suffering is physical.

Unfortunately, the doctor's diagnosis has a tendency to become permanent. The patient thinks, *Now I have it, I will always have it, and even if it goes away, it will someday come back again.* It becomes an intermittent but persistent permanency. This imprint into the memory bank, together with the imprint that it is physical and you can't do anything about it, triggers different emotional and bodily reactions or overreactions. When these two imprints are combined, it causes certain other emotional factors to come into play, giving rise to such symptoms as fear, anxiety, tension, and depression. In the case of a diagnosis of heart disease or cancer, there is a tremendous overreaction to the thought that you have something that is physical and permanent, and you can't do anything about it. The action or reaction is subconscious in origin because in the memory bank is the imprint or initial suggestion that only the doctor can handle this problem.

When the patient receives the imprint or impression that there is nothing the doctor can do and that death is waiting at the door, there comes a mental deterioration that causes a physical response. When the patient takes on the attitude that he has nothing to live for, the demise of the patient has begun. What is necessary is the change of attitude of the patient.

Several years ago, I consulted with a pathologist about the effects of cancer on the body. I was astounded to learn from him that after conducting over a thousand autopsies, he had concluded that the vast majority of the individuals examined didn't have enough cancerous cells to kill them. He couldn't understand how such minute cancerous tissues could create such destruction.

It has been my personal contention that people die of *the knowledge of cancer much more readily than of the disease itself.*

Recently I was asked to attend to a cancer patient who had just returned home from the hospital. He and his wife were packing to move into an apartment from their home which had just been sold. The home they were leaving was spacious, thus making it necessary for them to sell most of their furniture. My first visit was on a Friday, and most of the household furnishings had already been removed except for a few small items and two beds. My second visit was on the next day, Saturday, at their new apartment, where all the boxes were cluttering up their rooms. The wife and some of her friends were attempting to arrange some of the furniture in an orderly fashion and were in the process of emptying boxes. The patient was lying on the bed fully clothed and somewhat depressed because he was unable to help. We had good hypnotic sessions at which time a tape was made for his use between sessions. On the next day, Sunday, we had our third session and made a second tape for him. The patient had a complete change of attitude and was feeling much better. He was in excellent spirits and before I left, he stated, "I'm going to beat this damn thing." I left the next day, Monday, to attend a hypnosis convention in Chicago. I returned the following Sunday, just a week later, only to learn that he had passed away during my absence. The next day I had an extended visit with his wife and we discussed family attitudes in connection with the patient. I was not surprised to learn that she had a violent argument with her husband after my third visit on Sunday and in her anger she had remarked, "You're going to die anyway, so why not do it now and get it over with and save us all some grief?" Following that remark, the patient decided to die and willed his own death, and in *three* days he was dead.

There must be a continuing and ongoing education to make each of us believe that there is within us the capability to heal ourselves. When a person suffers a bone fracture, there is usually some extensive tearing of the tissues, rupturing of the blood vessels, and damage to the skin. After the fracture has been set and a cast placed to hold the bones in position, no further medical treatment is administered. It is the patient who thereafter repairs the fracture, mends the damaged tissue, and replaces the injured skin. We readily accept that this can be done and the body then heals itself. It is those areas in which we doubt our ability to heal that cause us the most concern. When we express the attitude that "I can't heal myself, so I must see the doctor," we leave ourselves open to stress and overreaction which, in turn, give rise to other symptomatic problems.

On the other hand, when after a complete examination, the doctor informs that patient that there is nothing physically wrong with him, this starts within the patient a whole new attitude. Since it isn't physical, it must be mental, and this carries a certain amount of stigma. Usually, there is a sigh of relief when something physical can be found; but when there is an indication that it is mental, there grows a feeling of belligerence. Many patients will move from one doctor to another, hoping to find a doctor who can find the problem because the patient "knows" that it is there. Since there are the normal expectations for the doctor to find the cause of the pain, a certain amount of stress and overreaction is created by the uncertainty when nothing physical can be found to give rise to the discomfort. This overreactivity then manifests itself into other symptoms, which will undoubtedly lead to a further spectrum of physical problems, i.e., ulcers, etc. So the advantage of hypnosis is in breaking up this confusion and adding logic to the thinking process. Since all emotional reactions or *programs of conduct* are the result of a thought process, then hypnotists need only to change the thought, and the conduct is modified.

Behavioral problems such as overeating, smoking, drug abuse, drinking, depression, emotional problems, phobias, sexual anxieties, learning disorders, family and/or work-related problems are all considered mental. These problems, being mental in origin, give rise to the delusion that we as individuals should be able to do something about them. Most of us have some education, either formal or work-related, and being so educated, we have a built-in implication that, since our problems are mental, we can correct them. Attempt after attempt has been made to make the necessary changes in our behavioral patterns.

And what is our first reaction to failure? Depression – we get angry and frustrated and feel guilty. Persons who have attempted to stop smoking or curb their excessive eating patterns end up with a feeling of self-condemnation. The negative thought is then created that one is either too weak or crazy. Isn't it strange that you can't stop doing something that you know is detrimental to your health? Now the imprints, impressions, or recordings are being stored in the memory bank of the brain for future reference. Each subsequent failure magnifies the problem. This, in turn, leads to further stress and overreaction and self-condemnation and subsequent withdrawal.

This condemnation continues up and until a visitation to the doctor's office when the patient states that he is too weak to handle his own problem, too nervous, has too many family troubles, and is too tired to think about them, thus harboring a guilt feeling for not being able to do what some other people have accomplished. The patient objects to paying the doctor for what he feels he should be able to do for himself. That's pretty much the standard reaction.

Little does the patient realize that making the changes is not a simple or easy task. Each of us uses thousands or millions of imprints every moment of our lives. Some are directed to the heart, lungs, eyes, hands, arms, legs, and all the other muscles and organic movements on an on-going basis without hesitation. In addition to using the past impressions and imprints of events long past, we continue to place in the brain a continuous flow of new imprints and impressions of events and ideas. So in the ordinary conscious thought process, we are attempting to unscramble the old unwanted suggestions or imprints, remove them, and install new ones. We find this process frustrating and sometimes impossible. When this situation becomes intolerable, we generally seek assistance from the physician who, in the ordinary course of his training, is unable to render any assistance. What is the procrastination time that an ordinary person such as a smoker or one who is overweight uses before he comes into the office? His automatic reaction is that he is fighting the fact that he has to pay someone for something he should be able to do for himself. It's always "one more time, just another try."

One of the most difficult tasks of the hypnotist is to break through the stubborn and resistant attitude of society and get rid of the negative feelings surrounding the use of hypnosis. The only way the individual attitude can be changed is by a learning process that leads to a change in one's reactivity. Learning the relaxing techniques reduces the need for a continuous flow of imprints and suggestions from the brain through the subconscious mind. Closing of the eyes shuts off incoming recordings into the brain. Adding new suggestions, thoughts, and imprints to the memory bank erases, interferes with, and overshadows the old impressions and imprints.

When someone reaches the "I can't" stage, he comes to the hypnotist for treatment and, to that patient, the treatment of hypnosis is the "pill," "medicine," or "surgery" that is required to heal himself. In other words, it is the thing that is going to cure him. The individual memory bank has retained the impression or imprint that hypnosis in itself is the cure. This is consistent with the history of mankind that someone else must administer "something" to effectuate a cure for those things that are not in the ordinary course of human events done by each of us. When it has been proven beyond a shadow of a doubt and *accepted*, then, will the cure be effectuated. When we *believe* that the body can cure any cancerous disease, then cancer may be no more of a problem than the common cold.

Everything works potentially for the person whose memory bank, subconscious mind, and brain are set up for it. Feed the information into it that it can be done, and it will be done without any conscious effort. The art of treatment using hypnosis is the art of conversation through use of the proper words.

We can use hypnosis by explaining what it is and giving it new meaning. Relate with it and it becomes more tangible. Add the critical faculty to the subconscious mind, and a whole new picture is created within us. The power of the subconscious mind channels all of the impressions, imprints, impulses, and events into the brain without the benefit of any analysis. Add reason, analyses, determination, and concentration, and the potential becomes unlimited. The resulting effect is automatic. The thought that precedes every physical movement is there in position just waiting to explode into action. At the designated time or event, the response automatically follows without the use of any conscious effort.

Life is a continuous cycle of changes, traumatic and otherwise. How we cope with these changes largely depends upon our attitude and its relation to the acceptance of these changes. Death, divorce, and financial problems are at the top of those traumatic changes and if we read these with the intention that they could make us sick, then the memory bank, i.e., the brain, is overloaded with negativity. Since life situations are always subject to continuous changes, we then ask ourselves, *"Is it the changes that make us ill or is it the way we handle these changes?"* It is neither. It is the attitude to the change and the negative overreaction caused by the events creating the changes. In the case of a heart attack or cancer or every other similar traumatic event, it is the intense overreaction. For heart attack victims, the traumatic questions are: "When will the next one come? Will it be fatal?" As to cancer, the questions are: "How long do I have? How long will I suffer?"

Negative overreaction is then channeled into the brain's computer data bank, the memory, and the body begins its deterioration process long before the disease manifests itself.

A change in attitude becomes necessary and absolutely vital for survival. A change in attitude becomes necessary for an increase in the quality of life. The reaction to a diseased state can be most significant and sometimes traumatic, and this action must be turned back and minimized but is not that easy to turn it back because it is so automatic, normal and natural. However, when the tide is turned in only one case and it becomes known through publications, it has a breaking effect. With more known successes, the automatic and normal acceptance of the "inevitable" will be cast aside with the change in attitude.

6

GENERAL TREATMENT

All behavioral patterns, also referred to as "programs of conduct," are the direct result of information stored in the brain. Whether the behavioral patterns are acceptable or unacceptable depends upon the nature of the information stored in the brain. The conscious awareness is the faculty by which this information usually is gathered. Remember that the conscious mind deposits this information into the brain after first analyzing it or filtering it. It can be accepted partially or totally, or it can be rejected partially or totally. During periods of emotional stress or suffering from traumatic events, or when the conscious awareness is not functioning at an efficient capacity, the subconscious mind then becomes the dominant factor of awareness. The more tragic or stressful the event, the deeper the state of hypnosis is needed. In the absence of rejection, the incoming information or suggestions are then automatically accepted as believable and true, and a pattern of behavior or programs of conduct then become stored in the brain's data bank with its full behavioral impact. This information is then utilized by the subconscious mind to create a behavioral response. These responses cannot be considered conditioned responses.

A conditioned response is one that is purposely created with the conscious awareness assisted by the subconscious mind. An example that we might all recognize is when a child comes home from school a little late and the mother states, "Your father wants to speak with you." The child, anticipating that he is to be disciplined, walks over to his father under stress and emotional anticipation. Then the father yells, "You stupid bum!" This remark is automatically accepted unanalyzed and remains in the child's brain. Repeating this remark compounds the suggestion of being dumb or stupid, and the child's behavioral pattern is now started in a negative manner. However, should the father, considering the same circumstances, shout out, "Congratulations! Your teacher said you were the best in the class!" a different behavioral response would result. This response would be positive.

As the conscious mind's efficiency is lessened due to stress, anxiety, depression, or traumatic events (just to name a few factors), the subconscious mind is increased up to a point where it becomes the dominant faculty. The information to which the person is exposed is then accepted, if not rejected, by the subconscious mind and deposited in the brain's data bank.

This information is referred to as the initial sensitizing event. Repetition of such events or events that are associated with them produce a greater anxiety in the person's mind, thereby creating a repetition of emotional discomfort associated with the initial sensitizing event. The information creating the initial sensitizing event and the associated or related events are then stored in the brain, which make a reality out of the person's confusing problem. As the feeling of reality increases in the person's mind, the greater the behavioral pattern is exhibited. The more real the fearful thoughts become, the more frightened the person becomes by those related thoughts. So instead of his feelings and thoughts being brought out so they can be openly scrutinized and discussed rationally, they are buried deep in the brain's data bank. Once buried, they then become the building blocks of the subconscious mind in creating a negative behavioral pattern. The result is an unacceptable behavior response without any conscious awareness. It then becomes an automatic response.

Remarkable results have been achieved through direct suggestions during hypnosis. These suggestions are positive in nature so that they can directly overcome the negative effects of the initial sensitizing event. Before we can assist the person or render any advice, we must first learn of his experiences and understand the influences these events have on the mind of the person. Therefore, the hypnotist must diagnose the detailed events stored in the person's data bank, together with their influence on the conduct of the person, in order to properly solve the disturbing problem.

There is a premise or *program* of conduct for the basis of each person's problem, and we usually must conduct a detailed and exhaustive search for that premise. Since we are searching for an event that created a sufficient threat or problem so that an area of anxiety was established in the person's mind, the place to begin is to return the person through age regression to the period when his disturbing problem first became noticeable.

These disturbing problems may be solved by bringing to light the initial sensitizing event and a review of the subsequent or associated events which gave reality to his feelings and behavior. Usually, unless this is done, the person will continue to be faced with his uncomfortable feelings and anxieties and become more confused. His problems will continue to grow, increasing his negative behavioral responses. However, with the use of the library technique more fully explained in Chapters 10 and 11, we can combine all related activities in one group without the detailed examinations of each event.

It was Dr. Josef Breuer who discovered that the simple recall of a traumatic experience from the past was responsible for removing the symptom. Dr. Lewis R. Wolberg then recognized the value of Dr. Breuer's dealing with the apparent cause of the symptom as differentiated from the direct removal of the symptom.

Once this initial sensitizing event has been revealed and discovered, the hypnotist and the subject can logically discuss the responsive patterns of disruptive emotional disorders or responses. Usually this will create a spontaneous resolution to the uncomfortable feeling and the anxiety state will diminish.

Since we know that the person's problems have their origin in past experiences, either physical or conversational, and that they have continued to exist in that person's brain, it now becomes apparent that we must commence an investigative process that will permit a search into the person's data bank through the use of the subconscious mind.

Before we drift too far astray here, let us backtrack for a moment into just what we are looking for and how to obtain it. First of all, each and every person's thoughts, ideas, wishes, desires, physical and mental experiences are gathered by the conscious and subconscious minds. The conscious mind functions primarily and the subconscious mind secondarily when the conscious mind is emotionally disturbed or temporarily occupied.

All of this gathered information is then stored in the brain's data bank. Any information which is of recent origin or of great importance or that which has been repetitiously deposited can be easily and readily recalled. The subconscious mind can recall deep-seated or buried information, and can utilize this information for instant and automatic body functions.

There are two ways to approach the removal of the person's uncomfortable feelings and disturbing problems: one way is to try to trace back through these experiences to the origin. This is called the Emotional Regression Technique. The other method is to determine, if possible, the person's first experience with his disturbing problem and then trace its development as it exists at the time of the commencement of the treatment.

This second method is called Emotional Development Technique. After the induction and deepening processes have been completed, some time should be used to develop a good rapport and select conversational words that will create a feeling of comfort and a calm, assuring atmosphere. This is most easily achieved by having the person recall amusing events in his life which stimulated his imagination.

The next step is to have the person identify the disturbing emotional feeling as it was experienced by him. These states of emotion or anxiety are very difficult to communicate in descriptive words. Usually during the first visit, the emotion will manifest itself by physical means, such as being fidgety, nervous hand movements, lack of expression, excessive talking, scratching, twitching, or uneven breathing patterns. Since the person's problems have had their origin in some event, by describing one's feelings, associated events will be revealed. Listen and learn from your subject, for he may provide an identifying clue as to the nature of events associated with his undesirable feelings.

The third step in this technique of emotional regression normally involves tracing the uncomfortable feeling back to its origin. This requires a step-by-step procedure recalling retroactively each event which has produced this uncomfortable emotional feeling which, in turn, has lent reality to his problem. The hypnotist should be persistent and patient in retracing these events back to their origin until a satisfactory explanation can be reached for the origin of his emotional problems.

Once these events have been traced back to the initial sensitizing events, a solution to the emotional and anxious problems is within reach. Since the initial sensitizing event was recorded and stored in the brain without the assistance of the conscious mind's analytical capabilities, it now rests upon the hypnotist to satisfactorily explain, rationally analyze, and minimize the importance of this event. The success of the treatment depends upon the efforts of the hypnotist in explaining in language readily understood by the subject and his ability to absorb the explanation. This treatment removes the anxiety from the person's mind and destroys the reality of the initial sensitizing and subsequent associated events.

If disclosing, analyzing, or explaining the initial sensitizing event does not relieve the person of this emotional problem, then one must look deeper into his first thoughts or impressions symbolizing death to himself. In this event, we find a more realistic threat to the person's health than has been previously ascertained. It then becomes absolutely paramount to clarify the lasting impressions of death, which is then only disguised by the other more manifested anxieties.

As explained in Chapter 2 in this book, hypnosis means entering a state of awareness dominated by the subconscious mind.

Having entered that state by means of induction and deepening techniques, the subject, through suggestion, can utilize his full subconscious potential. The suggestions and treatment of the hypnotist have a posthypnotic effect in minimizing the reality of the initial sensitizing event. Removing the reality in the initial sensitizing event, in most cases, is not adequate. The reality of all subsequent associated events that have perpetuated the emotional anxiety must also be considered.

Therefore, the logical step to follow is the Emotional Development Technique. Having developed the awareness of the initial event and having the knowledge of the nature of the person's emotional situation or fear, the solution seems to logically follow. Having regressed the person back from one event to another, we need only bring the person forward in time from one event to the next. As each event develops a logical explanation, rational discussion, and minimization should then be undertaken by the hypnotist. All responses to the events, especially fear, must be addressed and explained. Ridicule has no place in this treatment. All thoughts surrounding anxiety in the person's mind must be explained fully. With this, the person is ready for posthypnotic suggestions.

In all cases where fear is exhibited in connection with accidents, illness, or death, it is important to search into the deepest areas of the mind to disclose those thoughts of death or those symbolizing death. Once this thought or symbol has been established, it will be later associated with other experiences producing a real fear for survival. The hypnotist then, realizing this symbol, can remove the associated symbolic relationship on other events through posthypnotic suggestions. Once these disturbing thoughts are exposed to a rational analysis, the anxiety is removed from the mind by destroying the reality of such threats to the person's security.

A number of years ago, a patient complained of acute infection of the hands and arms which occurred at the time when he was tearing down a chicken coop. An examination revealed that he had acute dermatitis. A past history was taken, and the patient explained that a similar event happened some twenty years earlier when he had been working in an oil field. He stated that he had been poisoned by gas and had treatment for over two years before he completely recovered. In hypnosis, the patient explained that this illness had its onset when he had been working on an oil tank car and suddenly became dizzy and had the feeling that he would lose consciousness and fall into the tank car. As a result, his dermatitis started at once and he had to discontinue his work. However, further probing revealed that his initial sensitizing event occurred some ten years earlier. At that time, the patient observed a bird down in the bottom of a well and when he went down to rescue the bird, he became overcome by gas in the well. Just before he lost consciousness, he became aware of being dizzy and the smell of oil. The recalling of these events and minimizing their importance brought about an immediate relief from his dermatitis.

In another case, following breast surgery, a woman developed severe depression resulting in withdrawal and seclusion. She was unable to bathe herself, change her clothes, or share the same bedroom with her husband. Her depression became worse to the point where she could not continue her social activities. The entire illness developed during surgery. In hypnosis, the patient was regressed back to the surgery, where she stated that she had heard a nurse remark, "There is always cotton." At that moment, a picture had flashed through her mind of a girlfriend who had a breast removed. Due to complications, gangrene set in and further surgery was required, resulting in the entire wound being packed in cotton. Buried deep within the patient was a picture of herself someday being in the same predicament as her friend. The casual remark by the nurse caused that picture to become a reality immediately following the woman's surgery. The recalling of these events in hypnosis led to a complete recovery, and the entire depressive syndrome was removed.

A 46-year-old woman came to see me about her weight problems. She remembered as a child she was a little overweight; however, over the past twenty years, in spite of her serious endeavors to remain at a normal weight, she continuously added on several pounds each year. Her considered failure to maintain a proper weight finally got to her, and she suffered from depressive emotions. In hypnosis, she was regressed back to the age of three when she recalled being in a room with many adults. As this three-year-old child moved from one adult to another during the course of the day, she vividly remembered that each of the adults who were rather heavy was very nice to her, and those adults who were unpleasant or indifferent to her were rather thin. At that time, she remembered believing that in order to be a nice adult, one must be fat or heavy. As the years progressed, her need to be loved and to love was affected by her initial sensitizing event – that is, her being impressed with the belief that only fat people are nice. In hypnosis, this impression was analyzed and discussed, thereby removing its drastic effect. Immediately following the first session, she started to lose weight and she continued to lose weight until she reached her desired goal. Without reaching and analyzing her initial sensitizing event, all future attempts to lose weight would have ended up in failure, leading to increased depression.

Some twenty years ago, when I was bowling one evening, a doctor friend of mine approached me to discuss one of his patients. He informed me that this patient had an eighteen-year history of being in and out of various hospitals and sanitariums. On each return to the hospital, her arms from the fingers to the elbow were raw from a rash as though most of the skin had been rubbed away. Further investigation revealed that this was caused by the use of a strong detergent while washing white clothes by hand. I suggested hypnosis be used, but the doctor meekly admitted that he didn't know how to use hypnosis. The following day, the woman was hypnotized in the doctor's office and age-regressed to an event involving her washing clothes. Twenty years earlier she remembered that while she was separating the colored clothes from the white clothes prior to washing them, her little dog had crawled onto the white clothes and urinated on them. This event became so deep-seated within her that whenever she saw a dog lift its leg to urinate and observed the urine, she would go home and wash every piece of white clothing in the house. She would strip the beds, clean out the closets of all clean bedding and towels and any other white articles, and proceed to wash them by hand. This initial sensitizing event was discussed in hypnosis with the explanation that once the clothes are washed, all traces of urine are removed. One session was sufficient to bring about a complete recovery.

In each of these cases and in almost every case I have encountered, the problem is the repression of the initial sensitizing event. The theory of repression is the pillar on which the edifice of psychoanalysis rests. It is not always easy to elicit traumatic material from the subject. In some cases, he feels insecure because of the fear that his defenses are being stripped from him. Freud abandoned hypnosis because he was embarrassed that he could not hypnotize everyone and that the cures were only temporary. The best clinical use of hypnosis is to emphasize and use those methods which bring about greater awareness in the subject. Remember that the event eventually became the initial sensitizing event because the critical faculty of the conscious mind was diminished. In effect, the person had performed self-hypnosis and was in a state of awareness dominated by his subconscious mind.

Let's examine some of the cases already described:

When the woman saw her dog urinate on the clothes, she probably became emotionally upset and screamed, "I'll never be able to get those white clothes clean!" That remark became a posthypnotic suggestion, and the effect was carried for over eighteen years.

Consider the 46-year-old woman who had the weight problem since early childhood. She may have been shunned by some thin adult and as she was hugged by a fat person, she could have overheard a remark like this: "Stay away from that skinny, mean man." Although such a remark could have been made in jest, being of such a young age, she didn't realize it.

For the woman with the breast surgery, the casual remark that "there is always cotton" was sufficient to bring the deep-seated vision to the surface. This vision was "planted" in her memory bank while she apparently was under stress and suffering emotional anxiety during the period when she visited her friend in the hospital and saw her in an unenviable condition.

The patient with acute infection of the hands and arms had the origin of his initial sensitizing event while under severe strain and anxiety. This occurred when he was in the well and became unconscious. As his conscious awareness was leaving, his subconscious became the dominant factor and in his precarious predicament, the dizziness and smell of oil were associated with pending death. The fear of pending death can manifest itself in many ways. In this case, it showed its ugly head by causing the acute infection of the hands and arms.

In each case, a change must be made in the evaluation, and importance given to the initial sensitizing event as viewed by the subject. The hypnotist must avoid making direct requests for change and bring change about while emphasizing some other aspect of the event. Within the framework specifically designed to bring about a change in the evaluation of the event, the emphasis on the change should be diminished. The initial focus should be on the subject's gaining a degree of self-understanding of the event. This self-understanding is brought about by the hypnotist's step-by-step, however subtle, explanation that the initial sensitizing event is only one small incident in the entire life of the subject and therefore, only minute importance should be placed upon it. Yesterday's problems should be discarded with yesterday's garbage. They have served their purpose and should not be permitted to clutter up tomorrow's pleasures.

Over the years, I have found there is no symptom that is a manifestation of a symptom or mental illness that cannot be simulated by a responsive subject in the hands of a really capable hypnotist. One of the real values of hypnosis is the speed by which symptoms can be produced or relieved.

Since the symptom or the manifestation thereof can be simulated, this symptom or its manifestation can also be removed. Most initial sensitizing events are hypnotic in origin. That is, the person's conscious awareness has been diminished by some traumatic or emotional event, thereby making the subconscious awareness predominant. While the subconscious awareness is predominant, the person is in a state of hypnosis. The initial sensitizing event then becomes a posthypnotic suggestion in effect. The subject is really suffering from a posthypnotic syndrome. Years of continuous practice in the use of hypnosis has taught me that any emotional symptom created in hypnosis can also be removed in hypnosis. For example, mild or severe pain can be created in any part of the body and likewise it can be removed. Pain created by a sprained ankle can be removed. Pain or discomfort is a message from the injured organ, muscle, or tissue to the brain asking for assistance. Pain, like any other symptom such as love, hate, fear, taste, touch, etc., has no dimension, no substance or material being. These symptoms cannot be placed on a table for dissection or examination. They are related to the subconscious mind and can be "willed" away.

Recently, I had a young lady come in to see me because she wanted to quit smoking. Following one session, she had no further desire to smoke. During the initial session, I asked her, as I usually do, just why she desired to stay away from smoking. She related that her attending physician strongly recommended it and that since she was allergic to many things, this would help her combat her allergies. Her allergies were manifested by a twitching and irritation in her nose, watering of the eyes, and a coughing or choking spell. While she was in hypnosis, I told her I would gently touch her left knee with my finger, thereby causing the allergic attack, naming each symptom individually. I touched her knee three times, counting each touch, and within a few seconds she had an allergy attack. She was then told I would touch her right knee three times, causing the symptoms of the allergy attack to leave. Immediately following my touching her right knee, the symptoms left. She was a very good subject, highly suggestible and able to obtain a very deep state of hypnosis. Following the session, I remarked to her that she would not be able to get up from the chair she was sitting in nor be able to stand up. Try as she might, she could not get up out of the chair.

I appraised her as being a true waking somnambulist. She is a somnambulist because she enters a very deep state of hypnosis immediately. Her analytical portion of the conscious mind is limited in scope and ability. When I stated that she couldn't stand up, not having rejected the suggestion, she created a posthypnotic effect. Had the analytic portion of the conscious mind been active, she could rationalize that there was no reason why she couldn't stand. Following this reasoning, she would have easily gotten up out of the chair. According to my experience, many people fall into this category. Whatever statement she accepted as being absolutely true was ingrained in her subconscious. In addition, if she believed an event always created the same response, then she was locked into that response. In this particular case, if this girl believed she could not catch a ball thrown to her, she would not be able to hold the ball no matter from what distance it was thrown. Similarly, some people say, "I can't swim. If I go into deep water, I'll drown."

Generally speaking, we can classify people into three categories:

1. Those who are hypnotized and subjected to post-hypnotic suggestions.
2. Those who are exposed to traumatic or emotional events, where their conscious awareness is limited and their subconscious becomes the dominant factor. (In these cases, exposure to conditions or events and/or remarks will create posthypnotic responses.)
3. Those who experience waking somnambulism. (Believing in the spoken word or the acceptance of the response according to the event creates a posthypnotic response.)

In each of these categories, there are certain common denominators: acceptance, credibility, and expectation.

Every person always maintains the ability to accept or reject any idea, thought, or event within certain limitations. In the normal conscious state of awareness – that is, when the conscious mind is the dominating factor – acceptance is usually based upon credibility.

To accept something, one must rely upon its being believable. Since anything is possible in this state of awareness, we look at the probability of the truth of the matter. So in the conscious state of awareness, we accept the fact only if it is probably true. The acceptance is further limited depending upon the nature of the source of the information.

Suppose one day your car wouldn't start. So you lifted up the hood to examine the engine to determine what was wrong and a stranger came up to you. He said your generator needed to be replaced and your battery was worn out. The chances of your accepting these suggestions would be remote. However, if a mechanic informed you of the same thing after examining your car, you would readily accept this information and have the work done. This acceptance of the suggestion that the work had to be done was due to the status of the informer.

If you complained to your neighbor that you had stomach cramps and severe pain and he suggested you have your appendix taken out, you wouldn't immediately run to the hospital and have the operation. His suggestion would not be accepted or believed. However, if the same day you then were examined by a physician and he said your appendix was inflamed and had to be removed, you wouldn't hesitate to have the operation. Credibility, then, depends upon the probability of the matter being true. The conscious mind analyzes possibilities and probabilities before it accepts the information or matter.

Acceptance can be passive or active. Should the information or fact have little impact upon the future of the person, it is more likely that it will be accepted. If you were to walk up to a stranger who is smoking and suggest that he quit because he may contract lung cancer, in all probability he would remark, "I've been smoking for twenty years and I don't have it, so leave me alone." In his thoughts, lung cancer is for someone else and he will never get it, so that act of smoking has little impact on his future. However, if a doctor, now a person of authority, after an examination tells this same person that he is exhibiting signs of emphysema and it will get worse unless he stops smoking, the likelihood of the acceptance would increase.

Last, but not least, is the expectation. Things happen because there is the expected result of the happening.

A native of Africa is seriously ill with fever, so he calls in the witch doctor who enters his place of abode waving feathers and chanting and singing. Shortly, the fever subsides and the person is cured. We of the more civilized community may laugh and ridicule this practice. However, during World War II while I was serving in the Navy, I was called upon to administer assistance to those having headaches, back pain, stomach pains, seasickness, and other problems. For each patient, I had a special "pill" that was so strong that one was sufficient to cure all problems. They were unaware that the pills were salt tablets and all came from the same bottle. However, upon taking the pill, each was cured. They expected the pill to cure their problem, and it did. They all realized their expectancies.

Recently, I had a patient who came in because he wanted to quit smoking. During the session, he explained to me that he had been involved in an auto accident, had been seriously injured, and suffered severe pain in the left knee. While he was in hypnosis, I explained to him that I was in possession of a drug that was in the process of being tested and, although not yet approved for marketing, had produced amazing results in relieving pain. With his permission, I applied this lotion to his knee and immediately his pain was gone. I further explained that the lotion would remain effective for a period of about one week, giving his knee a chance to repair itself, and should the discomfort return, it would be noticeably less intensive. Two weeks later, he was still without pain. The lotion administered was nothing but hand lotion available at any drugstore. He believed my suggestion that the lotion was something special and accepted my suggestion that it would relieve his pain. Upon my administering the lotion, he expected something to happen. It all resulted in the realization of his expectations.

In hypnosis, the state of subconscious awareness, these three common denominators play a different role. The subconscious mind does not analyze. The suggestion is either accepted or rejected on an "as is" basis. The rejection must be actionable. That is, the subject must actively exert some thought or effort in casting it aside, refusing to carry out the terms of the suggestion, and rejecting its meanings. Unless this active effort is employed to reject the suggestion, the suggestion is automatically accepted. Passive acceptance is sufficient. During the interview, I always tell my patients that I need two things from them: (1) a desire to do or accomplish something and (2) the belief that it can be done. They come to see the hypnotist because they have a need and a desire to eliminate their problems, and they are there because they believe the hypnotist can help them.

The more successful the hypnotist becomes, the more the subject anticipates his problems will be relieved. The expectations of the subject are then realized by the hypnotic suggestions. When the hypnotist says to the subject:

> As I gently touch your right knee with my finger, it causes your knee to become numb and useless, even growing cold, numb, and useless ... and now the numbness is spreading down from your knee through each and every muscle, causing each muscle, nerve, and cell to become cold, numb, and useless. Now that feeling of coldness, numbness, and uselessness spreads up from your knee through each large and small muscle up to your hip, causing each muscle, nerve, and cell to become cold, numb, and useless. Your leg is now so limp, relaxed, cold, numb, and useless that you cannot lift it nor can you cross it over your left leg. The harder you try to lift it, the more it becomes heavier and useless. Try to lift it and you will find that you cannot.

When the subject tries to lift the right leg, he experiences a feeling of complete muscle relaxation to the point the leg feels cold, numb, and useless.

The suggestions made were not of such great importance to cause the patient or subject any concern and were passively accepted. The word "cause" was purposely inserted in the suggestion to create the necessary effect. The subconscious mind, not having analytical powers, failed to exercise any supervisory control over its acceptance. The subject is there for "treatment" and expects something to take place that will happen to him. The suggestion, not having been rejected, has been accepted. The credibility is "coined" into the suggestion by using the word "cause" and the subject realizes his expectations.

In all my suggestions, the terminology "cause and effect" is included. Whenever something is done, it causes something to happen and while it is being done, this something is happening:

> As I count backward from one hundred, each
> decreasing number <u>causes</u> you to relax more and more.
> And with each decreasing number, you <u>are</u> relaxing more
> and more. As each muscle relaxes, it touches the lower
> muscle, <u>causing</u> the lower muscle to relax and with each
> relaxing muscle, you are going deeper and deeper into
> relaxation.

Many hypnotists fail to receive a positive response from their subjects because they have failed to create the positive condition. Many hypnotists, even those who have practiced for years, are discouraged when the expected results are not achieved. I have heard hypnotists say, following their deepening techniques, "Now your hands are so relaxed that you cannot lift them up." When the subject is able to raise his hands, the hypnotist becomes confused and is unable to proceed in some cases. His explanation is that he was unable to get the subject deep enough to get a positive response. When attempting to create an adverse condition in any subject, such as heavy arms or heavy legs or eyes closing, a suggestion must be made to that effect. All adverse conditions must be specifically suggested and created, and every adverse suggestion created must be specifically removed. What you have done, you must undo.

Every person has experienced a large number of incidents, statements, and events accompanied by emotional feelings such as fear, pain, disgust, anxiety, love, hate, pleasure, guilt, etc. These incidents are stored away in the brain and are seldom brought forth on a voluntary basis. These events and incidents are brought from the depths of the memory bank upon the occurrence of a related or similar event. The recalling of the emotional events is involuntary and due to their rising uncontrolled emotions, we have the tendency to try to bury them as deeply as possible in our memory bank. We submerge them deeply so that we can never relive those traumatic responses. However, in most cases this is not possible; we seek some solution or remedy for our emotional conduct.

In using hypnosis, it is important to remember that we are dealing with the realities of the meaning of words. Hypnosis, by suggestion, deals with the transference and conveyance of ideas and understandings, and words are generally the means by which these ideas and understandings are conveyed. It then becomes evidently important that the language used by the hypnotist must be one that is readily understood by the patient or subject. When the person understands our language, we can readily arouse in that person parallels of our own mental thinking and processes so that the expected reaction may be achieved. Ideas and understandings can also be conveyed by means of extra verbal and nonverbal communications, and these means can help or hinder our endeavors.

During the interview, the hypnotist should go into the subject's employment and prior environment as these may be important in his interpretations of various words or phrases. It is important to remember that a person in a state of hypnosis interprets words literally and has very little, if any, sense of humor. Never try to impress the subject by using words or phrases in an attempt to convince the subject of your education. Rapport, which is essential in hypnosis, requires that you treat all subjects with dignity and respect.

Most persons believe that in using the word "sleep," we mean a condition of being relaxed, eyes closed, unaware of one's surrounding circumstances and conditions, such as being unconscious. A person in a deep state of hypnosis is not unconscious nor asleep as we normally refer to our experiences while in bed during the night. In order to eliminate unnecessary confusion, I never refer to or use the word "sleep" until I have completed all my induction and deepening processes. Before I use the word "sleep," I explain in detail just what I mean by using that word. For our purposes, my explanation is that "sleep" and "relaxation" are the same. Relaxation is a state of being where a person is resting quietly with the eyes closed and aware. For our purposes, the word "sleep" is also a state of being where a person is resting quietly with the eyes closed and aware. It must be further explained to the subject that at no time during the entire session, his awareness or consciousness is ever lost. With this explanation in advance, the need for further explanation will be eliminated, when following the session, the subject looks at the hypnotist and states, "You didn't hypnotize me because I heard every word you said and I was completely aware of everything around me."

This explanation not only assures the subject, but also relieves him of any unnecessary anxiety. It also makes it much easier for him to accept the suggestions that are made for his benefit.

7

INDUCTION

Induction is the method, modality, or technique employed by the hypnotist to transfer the subject from the conscious awareness to the subconscious awareness. In either state, the subject is fully cognizant of all surrounding circumstances and conditions, and at no time during the hypnotic session does the subject become unconscious or unaware, leading to the "I wasn't hypnotized" syndrome. In unusual cases and for exceptional reasons, the individual's awareness is reduced to a state of semiconsciousness. In cases where a major surgical procedure is necessary without the benefit of chemical anesthesia, this unusual state is required to relieve the patient of not only pain but anticipated apprehension during possible surgery.

In order to conduct and obtain successful induction results from the hypnotic session, several factors, such as imagination, rapport with the patient, and concentration must be given due consideration.

Imagination is the creation of an image in the mind by assembling related events, impressions and impulses contained within the memory bank. It is an indispensable element in producing hypnosis. The subject will only exhibit a suggested image if the components of the image are known to him from previous experiences, whether these are real, fictitious, or mere dream experiences. Imagination, therefore, is a vital component that favors suggestibility and susceptibility.

Rapport, in essence, is the relationship of trust and confidence established between the subject and the hypnotist or operator which is very important in the induction and maintenance of the hypnotic state. During the induction process, the subject's attention is focused in a directed manner inhibiting the response from outside stimuli and, as the inductive process progresses, the subject continues to lose his attention with outside surrounding circumstances, permitting his concentration to be focused to a greater degree on the suggestions of the hypnotist. A good rapport means easier induction. Transference, which is the establishment of a uniform thought process between the subject and the hypnotist, ensues when there is good rapport. As this transference becomes more concentrated, the analytical function is proportionately decreased, strengthening the connecting function that allows the hypnotist to establish relationships with any organic area. The subject's rapport with and attitude toward the hypnotist and induction techniques depend largely on the apprehension, nervous activity, expectations, and cooperation. While some subjects will accept any induction technique with little or no difficulty, others may react through passive-defensive reflexes. This acceptance or rejection of the hypnotic induction depends largely upon the subject's prior knowledge about hypnosis together with personal experiences.

Concentration reflex is the physiological basis of attention and without this concentration, deep hypnosis is unattainable. Expectation, which is the product of concentration reflex, is the foundation for this phenomenology. The expectant attention is directly related to the newness of the exposure of the subject to the hypnotic induction technique. The newer or more different the technique, the greater the concentrated reflex. The concentration reflex is largely dependent upon the functioning of the polysynaptic system, which is sometimes called preferential; for this system serves the preferences that control or rule the homeostasis of the human being. When a momentary excitation of a living cell is created or produced by suggestion while a patient is in a state of hypnosis, the resulting physiological process creating the change will remain much longer than the excitation caused by suggestion created while a patient is not in hypnosis. The excitatory process will last longer in the nervous system than in other cells of the body. When one induction technique fails to produce satisfactory results, the hypnotist should immediately proceed with a secondary induction. Likewise, when a method employed for deepening the state of hypnosis is not successful, a different method should follow. Any number of induction and deepening techniques should be attempted until the hypnotist is satisfied that the subject has obtained the required depth.

The personality trait of the hypnotist has a greater influence on the peculiarities of the dynamic structures that flow in the transference zone. This transference begins with the initial concentration developed by the hypnotist and conveyed to the subject. Suggestibility depends on the degree of concentration by the subject. The greater the anticipated result, the more successful the hypnotic session. A person enjoying good rapport and undergoing suggestion has the benefit of having the ordinary cortical activity inhibited in such areas not directly connected with the suggestions. There results a functional disconnection of the cortical activity.

Under ordinary circumstances, hypnosis cannot be induced unless verbal stimuli are employed from the beginning and throughout the entire session. Not only is what is said important, but how it is said, as each word or phrase represents a signal to the cerebral hemispheres. Cortical activity can be provoked or replaced by this signal, resulting in a change or modification of body activity.

The most important factor the hypnotist must utilize during the hypnosis session is the patient's thought process. The brain only responds to messages that the mind sends to the brain. The brain processes and programs these messages through the nerves, causing the body to respond to carry out the thoughts delivered by the mind. No physical activity is created unless the brain has received a message to do something. Once this message is received, the brain has no alternative but to carry out the message. The brain cannot overrule the mind. A person doesn't get out of a chair until there is a decision to get up. The person then walks in the direction that has been predetermined. Once the decision is made to do something, the brain will cause the body to respond in a manner that the thought is carried out. No thought, no response.

Action, reaction, or inaction during the hypnotic session is the result of certain stimulated suggested action started by the hypnotist. A state similar to hypnosis may occur following intense stimulus, causing the cerebral cortex to lose its controlling powers over the subcortical centers inducing cortical inhibitions. When a person becomes involved in a traumatic situation or is confronted with fear and stress, the ability to think clearly is affected, resulting in illogical conduct or action. It is during these periods of cortical inhibition that the conscious mind loses its control or effectiveness, permitting the subconscious mind to take charge. The subconscious mind, not having the power to analyze or sift the truth from fiction, feeds information, imprints, and impulses directly to the subcortical centers, causing them to act or react in accordance with the information delivered. Since all information delivered to the subcortical centers while in a state of hypnosis is true, whether in fact it may be false, an adverse behavior may result from this false fact being accepted, if not rejected. This enables us to better understand certain hysterical conditions and why strong emotional states can lead to conditions resembling hypnotic states such as amnesia. A strong negative emotion causes immediate cortical inhibitions.

When a person is stressed, upset, frustrated, fearful, or faced with some traumatic conditions, he enters into a state of unintentional or spontaneous hypnosis. A woman, whom I had seen several times for work-related stress, came in to see me all stressed out. Her husband almost lost three fingers in a construction accident and he was in pain. As she related to me the circumstances surrounding the accident, I interrupted her and said to her that she had another problem. I told her she couldn't uncross her legs and she couldn't. Then I said she couldn't talk and she couldn't. Her stress put her into a deep state of unintentional hypnosis and my suggestions, not being rejected, were, for her, true.

A gentleman who had been hired to finish constructing a 250-unit subdivision that had gone bankrupt, came to see me about his drinking problem. He sat on the couch and said that he could not relax until he spent four days on a beach in San Diego. He had his arms on the back cushions of the couch. I told him he couldn't take his arms off the back of the couch and he couldn't. I knew he was in hypnosis due to his stressful situation.

In an ideal hypnotic session, we have a relaxed subject, pleasant surroundings, good rapport, and a competent hypnotist. With this type of situation, good concentration and an expectant attitude will emerge, leading to a transference association. The hypnotist's words create a highly receptive vigil zone. The more concentrated the transference zone, the more easily are formed the temporary associations.

Directing the subject's attention and eye fixation will ordinarily result in eye muscle fatigue, blurred vision, and heavy eyelids. The spoken words acting simultaneously will enhance the speed with which the eyes will close and cause the identical and normal phenomena facilitating induction.

Experiments have proven that the eyes demand about one-eighth of the total body nervous energy for their proper functioning. Through directed concentration, reflex, and limiting the visual activity by having the subject close the eyes, the cortical excitation is dramatically reduced. The visual system is a highly defensive system and any stimulation to this system causes a defensive cortical inhibition, so it becomes extremely important for this system to be "shut down" during the hypnotic session to prevent emotional excitation.

There are basically two methods of induction from which all other techniques evolve:

1. Concentration on the visual system with proper suggestions, causing eye closure
2. Eye fixation with suggested concentration on relaxing other body muscles and areas, resulting in eye closure

In every induction technique or method, the result of suggestion is eye closure, relaxation, and developed concentration. There is at this stage an irradiation of the cortical inhibition extending to the motor analyzer. Inhibited motor analyzer indicates an impossibility of analyzing stimuli coming from the corresponding organs. A person in a state of hypnosis – that is, when the conscious mind is inhibited and the subconscious mind is the dominant factor – does not have the cortical ability to analyze the imprints and impulses formed by the suggestions of the hypnotist, resulting in weakened motor responses. The deeper in hypnosis, the less responsive the subject is.

There are four principal stages the subject passes through during the hypnotic session:

- Induction
- Deepening
- Therapy or suggestion
- Returning to the conscious state, sometimes referred to as awakening

The least important of these is the induction, although over the years it has commanded the most attention. The universal question is: "How do you hypnotize someone?" The standard answer for all those who practice hypnotherapy should be: "I don't. They hypnotize themselves by merely following my suggestions."

This, of course, would affect the ego of the hypnotist and probably take away some of his pride as a professional, however true it may be. But it is important to recognize, and I wish to reemphasize, that hypnosis is a subject-centered mechanism, rather than one that is a hypnotist-directed modality.

Everyone who has the ability to "think" and maintain a degree of concentration can be hypnotized. When the attention span is limited, so is hypnosis. With the use of concentrated effort, there is a narrowing of the perceptual fields – that is, the surrounding stimuli – resulting in a heightened attention span, leading to hypnosis.

When a subject enters the office, he exhibits a desire to be hypnotized and at the conclusion of the session, there is an expectancy of a cure for his negative behavior. Induction then becomes the realization of his expectancies and the greater his conviction of cure, the better the results obtained. The more concentration applied by the subject, the "deeper" into hypnosis he will journey until a maximum depth has been obtained. There is a direct relationship between the ability to concentrate and the depth obtainable in hypnosis. The more the subject is able to concentrate and follow the suggestions and images outlined and proposed by the hypnotist, the greater the obtainable depth and the faster the cure. It is very difficult, if not impossible, to hypnotize an imbecile, idiot, moron, infant, or senile person, due to their lack of attention and the inability to concentrate for a given period of time. The more intelligent the person is, the better a subject for hypnosis he is. At no time is anyone surrendering his mind to the hypnotist to manipulate it for the benefit or convenience of the hypnotist. Every suggestion, idea, or thought may be accepted or rejected by the subject, regardless of the depth of the hypnotic state.

Resistance, either active or passive, on the part of the subject manifests a lack of confidence in hypnotherapy or the hypnotist and without adequate motivation, the subject's problems cannot be solved. Whenever this resistance becomes evident, it is important to make the subject understand that you, the hypnotist, are aware of his lack of cooperation while still maintaining a search for the answer to his resistance. During the initial interview, a resistant subject will exhibit certain physical and/or emotional signs indicating his reluctance to fully cooperate in the induction procedure.

When such signs are present, the hypnotist should rely upon a method of induction that is slow and casual, permitting the subject to enter into a state of hypnosis without the realization that induction has occurred. When a person enters into a state of hypnosis – that is, when his awareness is dominated by the subconscious mind – three things always remain consistent:

1. An increased concentration
2. An increased relaxation
3. An increased susceptibility to suggestion

Increased susceptibility is due to appropriate motivation, belief, confidence, a favorable mental attitude, and expectation, which differentiates hypnosis from force and persuasion.

There are as many hypnotic induction techniques as there are hypnotists. These methods of induction will vary entirely from recognized procedures or will be modifications of universally employed techniques involving stimulation of any one or all the senses. Such procedures usually fall within two general categories:

1. Slow induction used during therapeutic sessions
2. Instant or rapid induction used for entertainment or emergency and hospital use.

Since most of the hypnotist's time will involve treating the subject for behavioral modification or symptom removal, several slow or disguised methods should be mastered by the hypnotist.

Under ordinary circumstances when a subject or patient calls the office for an appointment for a hypnotic session, he has already exhausted all other means of securing relief from his negative behavior patterns. He has lived with his problems long enough and is ready to shed them and eager to begin his hypnosis treatment. However, the longer he is kept waiting for the appointment, the more apprehensive he becomes. All attempts should be undertaken to have the sessions commence within a twenty-four hour period after receiving the request for an appointment.

Upon completion of the interview and before the initial induction attempt, the subject should be administered at least two "suggestibility tests." These tests have a twofold purpose: first, to apprise the hypnotist as to the active or passive resistance of the subject and second, to put the subject at ease and remove some of the unnecessary tension and apprehension at being hypnotized.

Anticipate that every subject, regardless of his prior experiences with hypnosis, harbors some passive resistance and remains reluctant to the idea that someone is going to delve into his thought processes by some means unknown to him.

I have found that the following language is quite acceptable to most subjects:

> I would like to have you stand up, and I am going to give you three tests just to see how well you are going to respond. These are only tests and I am not going to try to hypnotize you.

Since these are only tests, there is no actual reason for the subject to anticipate anything more than a testing program. With this in mind, there is some relief from tension and anticipation.

The first test is the Swaying Test. The subject is asked to look at a picture or something on the wall while the hypnotist positions himself about two feet behind the subject and places his hands on the subject's shoulders, saying:

> I want you now to lean back into my hands.

The subject is permitted to lean back about ten inches with some tension on the arm muscles, so the subject feels secure. At that point, the subject is pushed slightly forward so he stands erect again. This should be repeated two or more times in order that the subject is assured that the hypnotist is capable of holding him up in a leaning position.

Standing behind as close as possible without touching the subject, the hypnotist extends his arms straight out over the shoulders of the subject with the fingers slightly turned in and in front of the subject's eyes as far as possible. With the hands remaining outstretched in this position, the hypnotist says:

> I want you to look at my fingers and as I draw them back, you will feel an invisible force push you back. And

the closer my fingers come to your eyes, the stronger

the force, causing you to fall backward into my arms.

Now the hypnotist slowly pulls his hands back toward the subject's eyes, continuing with the following language:

Feel the force beginning to push you back, back,

and growing stronger and stronger ... pushing you back

... back ...

In 90 percent of the cases, the subject will fall back into the arms or against the shoulder of the hypnotist. Make sure that your feet are planted firmly so the leaning subject does not cause you to lose your balance and fall, causing injury. The more resistant the subject is, the less likelihood that he will fall backward but there will be a noticeable movement of the shoulders. The time devoted to this test should not exceed one minute.

The next test is the Arm Relaxing Test. The hypnotist or instructor places his hands about ten inches in front of his waist, palms up, and asks the subject to place his hands on the hypnotist's hands, palms down. The subject is then asked to concentrate and relax all the shoulder and arm muscles so that when the hypnotist pulls his hands away, the subject's arms will fall limply at his sides. This is done two or three times to obtain and ensure complete relaxation. The noncooperative or resistant subject may have to be encouraged several times by saying:

You are doing pretty good, but I'm sure you can

relax those arms even more.

Always compliment your subject by saying:

You're doing fine. That's pretty good.

As you stated earlier that there would be three tests conducted and since there has been no attempt to hypnotize the subject during the first two tests, the tension or passive resistance has now been minimized. The third test is an induction technique which may be any one of the methods that the hypnotist feels appropriate for the subject. In order to obtain the best and fastest results from your induction methods, do not advise the subject that you are now going to hypnotize him.

There are three basic steps that should be followed while proceeding with the slow induction technique:

1. An explanation should be given to the subject of just what you are going to do.
2. After the explanation, the induction procedure should commence.
3. Suggestions of relaxation should be directed to the subject.

FINGER INTERLOCKING INDUCTION

The subject is told that this test is to measure his concentration and response to various suggestions. He is not told that this is an induction procedure or he will set up a passive resistance, even though he may be a very willing subject for hypnosis. The hypnotist demonstrates with the subject the various arm positions until the overhead position is reached, at which time the hypnotist lowers his arms to his sides. The induction proceeds as follows:

Extend your arms straight out from your shoulders,

place your palms together, interlace your fingers, turn

the palms outward, and raise your arms up and over

your head just as high as you can, palms facing upward

and fingers interlocked.

The hypnotist now drops his arms to his sides and steps in front of the subject not more than two feet away. Looking into the subject's eyes, the hypnotist continues:

I want you to look into my eyes. I am going to count from one to five. And as the numbers increase, it causes your fingers to lock tighter and tighter. And when I reach the count of five, your fingers will be locked together so tight that you will not be able to separate them or take them apart.

One. Your fingers are beginning to lock together tight, tight ... tight and tighter. Your arm muscles are beginning to grow tired and maybe rigid ... more tired.

Two. Your fingers are locking tight, tight, very tight. Arm muscles growing more and more tired. Now your eyes are growing tired and your eyelids are beginning to relax in order to close and ease your tired eyes.

Three. Your fingers locked together tight, very tight ... arm muscles tired and growing stiff and rigid, holding up your arms. As your fingers lock together tighter and tighter, they cause your eyelids to relax more and more, pulling them down so they close and ease your tired eyes.

Four. Now your fingers are locked so very tight. Eyes so very tired ... and your eyelids relaxing and closing. Let your eyelids relax and feel them closing, relaxing and closing, closing, closing, and closed. Let them close.

If the subject's eyelids are not closed by this time, then ask the subject to close the eyelids. Continue as follows:

> Five. Now your fingers are locked together so tight that you cannot separate them. The harder you try to separate them, the tighter they stick together. Try to separate them, but they will not separate. You cannot separate them, so stop trying.

As soon as you realize the subject is having some difficulty trying to separate his fingers, ask him to stop trying. Don't let him try too long. As he is trying to separate his fingers, gently slide your hands up his arms, grasp his wrists and state as follows:

> I am going to hold your wrists and lower your arms and as your arms are lowered, it causes the arm muscles to relax and let go. Feel them relaxing as I gently lower your arms and as the arm muscles relax, it causes your eyelids to progressively relax more and more.

Bring the arms down about chest high and hold them there as you continue as:

> Let your eyelids relax, and now let that relaxation flow from your eyelids down into your cheeks and then down to your neck. Feel that relaxation flow across your shoulders and down your arms. Let those arms relax.

Lower the hands all the way down to the sides of the subject and let go of one of his arms.

> Every word that I speak causes you to relax deeper and deeper, always feeling more comfortable and more relaxed.

Eye Fixation Induction

The subject should be comfortably seated in a chair or a recliner with his legs uncrossed and his arms at his sides so the fingers do not touch. In cases where it is necessary, the subject may be resting in bed. The subject is then directed to select and look at a spot on the ceiling, indicating a point that requires the subject to raise his eyes so it would appear that he is looking over the forehead at the selected point. Looking at the selected point in this position automatically causes his eyes to become tired.

With the subject in this position, the hypnotist may start his induction as follows:

> Keep your eyes fixed on that spot on the ceiling and as you do so, I want you to concentrate on relaxing your shoulders ... your shoulders relax ... let your shoulders relax ... relax each and every muscle and let go ... allow the feeling of relaxation to settle into each and every muscle ... and while these muscles continue to progressively relax, let that feeling of relaxation flow down your arms, causing each and every muscle of both your arms to relax and let go ... relax ... let your arms grow limp and relaxed ... as you continue to look at the spot on the ceiling, feel your eyes growing tired ... progressively more tired as you continue to gaze at that spot on the ceiling ... as your body continues to relax, it causes your eyelids to start relaxing, just as though they want to close and ease your tired eyes ... let your eyelids relax and let go ... feel your eyelids want to close and ease your tired eyes ... feel the relaxation settling down into your legs ... let those leg muscles relax ...

make them relax ... and as you continue to sit in that chair ...

(or "lie in that bed")

... each passing moment causes your arms and legs to progressively relax more and more ... so just let your eyelids relax and ease those tired eyes ... feel those eyelids want to close ... feel them closing ... closing ... closing ... closing ... closed and keep them closed.

The eyelids should now be closed and the subject showing signs of physical relaxation. However, in the event that the eyelids are not closed, then just continue with a cycle of suggestions of relaxation directed to the arms, legs, shoulders, and other parts of the body until closed eyes are obtained.

PALM INDUCTION

The subject should be seated in a chair with legs uncrossed and the arms should be positioned at the sides in a relaxed manner. Place your hand about three feet above the forehead, palm down, so the subject is required to raise the eyes in order to look at the palm. Holding the hand in this position, state:

I want you to look into the palm of my hand. By placing my hand in this position, I am suggesting relaxation. And each and every time that I suggest relaxation, you do relax pleasantly and deeply. Each subsequent time you relax, you do relax quicker and deeper than the previous time. As you look at the palm of my hand, this causes your eyes to grow tired, causes your eyelids to grow heavy, heavy with relaxation. As I lower my hand closer to your face, it causes your eyes to

> become tired, and your eyelids heavy with relaxation.
> And the closer my hand gets to your face, it causes your
> eyes to become progressively more tired and your eyelids
> progressively more relaxed. And before my hand touches
> your forehead, your eyelids do close and you do relax
> pleasantly and deeply, feeling very comfortable and very
> pleasant.

Once you have explained to the subject what is about to happen, very slowly lower the hand toward the eyes, continuing as follows:

> Let your shoulders relax. Now I want you to send
> that relaxation down both of your arms. Let those arm
> muscles relax and grow more and more comfortable. Let
> your chest muscles relax. And feel with each and every
> breath you take that your relaxation is growing deeper
> and deeper. So why not just let yourself relax? Feel your
> eyes grow tired, eyelids heavy with relaxation. Now let
> your legs relax. Let them grow limp. Eyes growing more
> and more tired, and eyelids heavier and heavier with
> relaxation. Feel them closing … let them close. Eyelids
> relaxing and closing … relaxing and closing … closing
> … closing closed.

Just before the hand touches the forehead, the eyelids should be closed. In the event that it appears they will not be closed, then just ask the subject to close his eyes. The psychological effect of the lowering of the hand is that the hypnotist is "occupying" the space of the subject. The only measure or method of retreat is to close the eyelids and shut out the outside stimuli or the crowding effect of the lowering of the hand. Having so retreated, the subject has entered into a light state of hypnosis so the posthypnotic suggestions and deepening techniques may begin.

TWO-FINGER INDUCTION

The subject is seated in a comfortable position with both feet flat on the floor and hands resting on the arms of the chair or on the thighs of his legs in a position so the fingers on one hand do not touch the fingers of the other hand. Make a fist with the right hand and then extend the first two fingers, continuing to hold the thumb and last two fingers in a clenched position. Hold the clenched hand in a position about fifteen inches in front and above the eyes so that it is necessary for the subject to raise his eyes, looking slightly above the forehead. With the hand remaining so positioned, start as follows:

> I want you to keep looking at my two fingers. And in a moment, I am going to lower and raise them five times. Each time as I lower them, I am going to count and as the numbers increase, it causes your eyes to become progressively more tired and your eyelids progressively more relaxed. So that by the time I reach the count of five, your eyelids do close and you do relax pleasantly and deeply.

Having explained what you are going to do, you then start very slowly lowering your hand to about the position of the subject's chin. Count *"one"* and then raise your hand back to the original position. Each time you lower your hand down to the position of the chin, continue counting until the number five has been reached.

While you are lowering and raising the hand, the following language should be spoken in a very easy and pleasant manner:

Let your shoulders relax ... let your shoulders relax ... allow your arms to relax ... make them relax ... with each and every breath that you take, your relaxation is growing deeper and deeper ... just breathe free and easy ...

One ... let your legs relax ... allow your legs to grow limp with relaxation . . . concentrate and relax those leg muscles ... each passing moment as you sit in this chair causes you to relax even deeper and deeper ... and with each passing moment, you are relaxing progressively more and more ...

Two ... allow your eyes to grow tired ... feel them growing misty and more and more tired as you continue to look at the ends of my fingers ... as your body continues to relax more and more, it causes your eyelids to become heavy with relaxation ...

Three ... now your eyelids want to close and ease your tired eyes ... feel them beginning to relax and close ... let them relax ... shoulders, arms, and legs continue to relax more and more as you continue to look at the ends of my fingers ...

Four ... eyes growing more and more tired ... eyelids heavier and heavier and heavier with relaxation and now closing ... closing ... closing ... closing ... let them close ... and closed ...

Five.

The hypnotist's attention should at all times be directed to the eyes of the subject so that any fluttering of the eyelids will be immediately noticed. When this occurs, more attention should be concentrated on causing the eyelids to become heavier and heavier with relaxation. Should the eyelids close before the count of five is reached, the hypnotist should continue the count without any further suggestion of relaxation. However, in the event that it should appear the eyelids are not going to close by the time the number five is reached, the subject should then be firmly instructed to "close the eyes and relax."

Remember that the closing of the eyelids automatically shuts down one-eighth of the body function, causing an immediate state of light hypnosis. Whenever it appears that there is some resistance to eye closure in the subject, the hypnotist should be firm and insist that the subject close his eyelids. In any induction procedure, when it appears that the subject is reluctant to close the eyelids or exhibits any apprehension, the request to close the eyelids should be in a firm but somewhat mild manner until the eyelids are closed. In some very reluctant cases, it may be necessary to repeat the request several times before the subject is willing to close the eyelids.

Always be insistent and take charge of the session.

INSTANT OR QUICK INDUCTION

This induction is not recommended for therapeutic purposes as it has a tendency to enhance the apprehension and anxiety of the subject. In some cases, it may be used during subsequent sessions where the subject has continually expressed doubt in being hypnotized or in cases where adequate depth is not obtained during the first and second sessions due to the non-cooperation of the subject.

The hypnotist should stand not more than two feet away facing and looking into the eyes of the subject and state:

> Just continue to look into my eyes and I want you to
> understand that you will be able to hear, see, and do

anything that you would like to do during this session.
All you have to do is follow my simple instructions and
you can enter into a pleasant state of hypnosis. Take a
deep breath and hold it ... hold it ... now slowly, very
slowly exhale it and let yourself relax. Now take a
second deep breath very slowly and hold it ... hold it ...
and very slowly exhale.

As the subject is asked to take a second deep breath, the
hypnotist lifts both of his hands above the subject's head. During the
exhaling, one hand is lowered behind the head and the other hand is
lowered in front of the head, passing close to the subject's eyes. The
hand behind the head is held near the neck without touching the
subject while the hand in front is held about shoulder high. With the
hypnotist's hands in this position, the hypnotist continues:

Now I'm going to count down from five to one and
when I reach the count of one, you will go quickly into a
deep state of hypnosis, deeper than you have ever gone
before.

Five ... Four ... Three ... Two ... And one.

At the count of *"one"* the hypnotist, using the hand behind
the neck, pulls the subject's head forward, simultaneously saying
in a very loud and commanding voice:

Sleep.

The head is pulled forward so that it rests on the hypnotist's
shoulder. Immediately, as though in a continuous motion, the head
is gently rocked from side to side in a rotating manner while,
massaging the neck muscles, the hypnotist continues:

Let those muscles relax and go deeper and deeper
asleep ... relax those neck and shoulder muscles ... feel
them relaxing ... now as I count, you are going deeper

and deeper ... feeling more relaxed and more comfortable.

Ten ... going deeper and deeper into relaxation ...

Nine ... feel those arms growing limp ...

Eight ... eyelids becoming more and more relaxed ...

Seven ... nothing bothers you ... nothing disturbs you ... let yourself relax ...

Six ... back muscles relaxing ...

Five ... you are in perfect balance and leg muscles growing strong and sturdy ... holding you erect and comfortable ...

Four ... your body continuing to relax ... progressively relaxing with each movement of my hand on your neck ...

Three ... each and every time I suggest sleep you will go quickly and soundly asleep ... always feeling more comfortable and more relaxed ...

Two ... whenever I suggest sleep, it causes your eyes to grow tired and your eyelids very relaxed and they will close ...

One ... each and every time you relax and sleep, you sleep deeper than the previous time.

To deepen the state of hypnosis, the subject may be asked to count backward from ten. During the counting procedure, the hypnotist should continue suggestive relaxation of the various muscles of the arms, shoulders, and legs. As an alternative method of counting, the subject may count from fifty to forty-five to forty, etc. When using the numbers as a deepening technique, always have the subject count backward. Use the forward count for awakening. Be consistent.

Stress Removal Induction

This technique is a little different because it allows the hypnotist to vary the subject's psychosomatic awareness both externally and internally, and allows the individual to dissolve the most vulnerable tension area, thereby allowing the entire body to relax.

The subject should be comfortably seated in a chair with feet uncrossed and placed on the floor. The hypnotist states:

What area or part of your body do you now find or usually find to be the most tense?

(The subject responds.)

Now describe in one or two short terms the most relaxing experience you have ever had in your life.

(The subject responds.)

I am going to have you go through a little exercise with me, so just lower your head and bury your chin down on your chest and close your eyes. Now count down from five to one slowly and very quietly, just loud enough for me to hear you while you are thinking about that most comfortable and relaxing experience ...

Lift up your head ... now put it back down on your chest and again count back down from five to one ... and this time as you do so, concentrate on relaxing that tense and stressful area of your body ...

Once again lift up your head ... and now lower it down to rest on your chest ... once again, count backward from five to one and let the thoughts of the most comfortable experience release the tension in the stressful area of your body ...

When all the stress and tension is removed, then just let your head rest on the chest and regard yourself in complete relaxation ...

Picture visually this most relaxing experience while working out the tenseness in your body. You may notice the circumstances around you and that my voice is soothing and relaxing. And as you become aware of these things, it causes you to go deeper and deeper into relaxation. And now as you continue to think about the most relaxing experience, it causes you to feel the most relaxed sensation that you have ever experienced ... so let the relaxed feeling take over your body and relax.

When I say the word relax, you will allow your attention to remove and dissolve the tension and stress in the problem area. And the rest of your body will follow in a beautiful process of complete relaxation. Enjoy this peaceful state of relaxation ...

Now think of the most beautiful and positive thing that you now have going for you at this moment of your life ... you find yourself feeling alert, refreshed, and bright ... and that wonderful and positive feeling that you have going for you will continue to be with you and will continue to carry you through the coming months.

GROUP INDUCTION

The subjects should be comfortably seated, facing the hypnotist who is standing about six feet in front of them. These subjects are now instructed to look into the eyes of the hypnotist, even though the hypnotist is not returning the glance. The hypnotist then looks into the eyes of one of the subjects and then slowly moves his glance until he has looked into the eyes of each subject's eyes once. Now, as the hypnotist slowly looks into the eyes of each subject from one to the other, he very slowly lowers his head and very slowly closes his eyes. The hypnotist then very slowly raises his head, opening his eyes. The process of looking from one subject to another while lowering and closing the eyes continues until the feeling of relaxation and eye closure are transferred to each of the subjects. As each subject's eyes close, then the hypnotist concentrates on the remaining subjects until all of them have closed their eyes.

The arms of the subjects are lifted and held extended straight out shoulder high. The hypnotist then snaps his fingers about six inches in front of the subjects' faces, causing, in most cases, the eyelids to open. Should the eyelids open, then the hypnotist gently lowers his hand from the subject's forehead down to the chin, gently saying, "Relax and deep sleep." When the eyelids are closed, then the subject's arm is lowered with the suggestion of complete relaxation.

This procedure is then carried out from one subject to another until the process has been completed with each subject.

PRINTED CARD INDUCTION

Cards should be printed in advance so the lettering is uniform and legible. Pass the cards out to the subject or subjects (as the case may be) with the printing face down. When all the cards are passed out, instruct the subject or subjects to turn the cards over and follow the instructions. Each card is printed as follows:

1. Trust me.
2. Follow my instructions.
3. Let your chin fall to your chest.
4. As you close your eyes, let the card fall from your fingers.
5. SLEEP

When the card falls to the floor, the hypnotist continues:

Now that your eyelids are closed, let that pleasant feeling of relaxation enter the forehead and gently flow down through each and every muscle of your whole body until it touches the end of your toes. Imagine the feeling of having a pleasant, warm, soothing liquid flowing down from the top of your head, gently touching your skin as it seeps down to your feet, causing every little cell in your whole body to just let go and relax.

NONVERBAL INDUCTION

The subject is seated in a comfortable position in an upright chair with the hypnotist standing behind the chair. The hypnotist then places his hands on the shoulders of the subject, requesting that the subject take a deep breath and slowly exhale. This should be followed by another deep breath and again slowly exhaling.

The hands are then removed from the shoulders and held waist high behind the subject about six to ten inches from the subject. Without touching the subject, the hypnotist then raises and lowers his hands in a circular massaging motion behind the subject. As this motion continues, the hands are slowly raised so the motion moves upward from the lower back to the shoulders. Continuing this motion, the hypnotist starts with the massaging of the lower back and then works his way up to the forehead.

At this point, the hypnotist then lowers his hands behind the shoulders of the subject and slowly moves them up to the top of the head in a manner that would appear as though he were pushing the air against the head, causing it to fall forward so the chin rests on the chest of the subject.

The massaging process is continued until the head falls forward and the eyelids are closed.

TEMPLE TOUCHING INDUCTION

The hypnotist sits next to the subject and places one hand behind the subject's neck and the other hand above the forehead in a manner permitting the hypnotist to place the thumb on one temple and the fingers on the other. The hypnotist says:

Concentrate on the point of your forehead that I am touching and feel that area growing warm, pleasantly warm, as I continue to hold my fingers on your forehead. Let that warmth flow down through your whole body, causing the muscles to gently relax. As each muscle relaxes, it causes the lower muscle to let go. And relax so that each muscle, gently relaxes from your forehead all the way down to your toes.

(Remove fingers.)

Each and every time that I touch your forehead, it causes your body to progressively relax deeper and deeper.

(Replace fingers.)

As those muscles relax, it causes your eyelids to become relaxed and closed.

The fingers are removed from the forehead before the hypnotist starts the sentence, "Each and every time that I touch …" and following the sentence the fingers are replaced. The hands remain stationary. It is only the fingers that are moved, so that there is very little movement and very little distraction for the subject. This may be repeated several times during the induction. The hypnotist continues:

> Now let that relaxation seep down deep into each
>
> and every muscle … let those muscles relax … let go …
>
> that beautiful feeling of relaxation flowing down deep
>
> into your body … eyelids growing heavy with relaxation
>
> and closing … closing … closing.

FINGER ON HEAD INDUCTION

The subject is seated in a straight-back chair with the hypnotist standing in front of him. The hypnotist's right hand is clenched into a fist except that the forefinger is extended. The finger is held in front of the subject about eye level and twelve to fifteen inches in front of the subject.

While the hypnotist proceeds with the following language, the finger is slowly raised over the head and brought to a rest on top of the head:

> Look at my finger and continue to keep your eyes on
>
> my finger as I slowly raise my hand above your head.
>
> When my finger is out of sight, imagine that you can
>
> look through the top of your head and see my finger.

(Now slowly start to raise the hand until the finger is rested on top of the head and continue with the following language.)

Just keep looking at my finger as it continues to
raise up … up … up … eyes growing tired … tired …
tired … eyelids relaxing … relaxing … relaxing.

(Finger is on top of the head.)

Take one deep breath and count backward from
three to one as you exhale and let your eyelids relax and
close. Now let that relaxation flow down through your
entire body, causing you to feel pleasantly comfortable.

Disguised Method of Iinduction

The basic principle of inducing hypnosis in a disguised or
indirect manner is to keep the subject uninformed as to the true
nature of hypnosis. Permit the subject to maintain his misconceptions of hypnosis and the subject will remain unaware of
his surrounding circumstances. Avoid the use of associated terms
such as "hypnosis," "sleep," or "trance."

Have the subject seated in a comfortable position or if
necessary, have the subject lie down on the couch or bed, removing
all unnecessary disturbances such as other members of the family,
pets, or music. Request that the eyelids be closed and that the subject
think of relaxing images or pictures. Proceed now with the
Progressive Relaxation Technique (outlined in Chapter 11) where
the subject is relaxed from the forehead down to the toes.

When it appears that the subject is satisfactorily relaxed,
then continue as follows:

Place both of your hands, palms down, on your
thighs so that they are gently touching the material you
are wearing. Don't press down. Just let your palms
touch the material ever so lightly. Concentrate on the
palm of your right hand and imagine that you are able to

feel the strands of the material as they weave in and out, forming a particular pattern. As you concentrate, the skin on the palm of your right hand becomes more sensitive and you may even be able to distinguish the various strands. Think about it and let your hand absorb the feeling of the material. As you continue to concentrate, you become aware that your right hand is growing more sensitive and that you can even feel the circulation of the blood against the palm of your right hand. And you may even feel the pleasant and comforting pulse of your heart as it circulates this life-maintaining process. As you continue to think about this circulation, you feel more and more satisfied and relaxed, knowing that everything is working just as you would expect it to. Every pulse and every heartbeat cause the right hand to become progressively more relaxed. So why don't we just let that hand grow absolutely relaxed as we move over to the left hand?

Direct the subject's attention to the left hand and follow a similar language pattern as used on the right hand, slightly varying the words. When the left hand is relaxed, then continue as follows:

Now that the right hand has completely relaxed and all the tension and restriction have been removed from the muscles, you can concentrate and begin to feel the circulation of the blood through the channels as it moves from your hand up to your elbow and back down again. Concentrate and experience that pleasant feeling, causing the arm to further relax and relieve all tension and restriction. Now feel that circulation all the way up to your right shoulder as it returns down to the palm of your right hand, further relaxing all of the muscles of your whole right arm. You know the circulation is always continuing throughout the entire body in an ongoing experience, so feel the circulation flowing from your right arm across your shoulders and down the left arm, relaxing each and every muscle that it touches. You may now be aware of the pleasant feeling flowing from your right palm up your arm across your shoulders and down the left arm into the palm of your left hand and returning up and back to the right palm. Feel that pleasant and continuous circulating flow of relaxation as it passes from one palm to the other and back again, progressively relaxing each and every muscle in both of your arms, causing them to become so relaxed that you hardly know they belong to you, let alone care. Let them relax. The right arm is growing progressively more and more relaxed, and you have the feeling it is so relaxed you cannot lift it up no matter how hard you try. Even your thoughts of lifting the arms cause your arms to become more and more relaxed, so totally relaxed, you cannot lift them. And the harder you try, the more relaxed they become.

I have used the disguised or indirect method in the induction process for cancer and terminally ill patients successfully. Seldom have I referred to my initial induction as hypnotherapy as there would have been a reluctance to "experiment" with such methods. The general conception of these terminally ill patients is that if the best medical treatment cannot cure their ailments, there is no other hope.

Little do they realize that within each and every patient is the potential for an absolute cure. Acceptance and expectation will normally lead to an improved quality of life. After seven or eight treatments, one of my cancer patients turned to me one day and asked, "Say, are you hypnotizing me?" I readily admitted it, to which he replied, "I thought so."

HYPNOTIC INDUCTION TECHNIQUE

A dentist should take a few moments of his time to explain to his anxious and apprehensive patient that glandular activity and tension greatly increase the sensitivity of all nerve endings and since this sensitivity is increased with tension, the reverse is also true – that this sensitivity can be equally decreased with a relaxed patient. The more relaxed the patient is, the less sensitivity. And since the dental work must be done for the benefit of the patient, it seems only logical that this work be done with as little discomfort as possible.

Before starting the relaxation process, the dentist or the dental assistant should request that the patient adjust his position in the chair so as to be as comfortable as possible, with legs uncrossed and hands placed on the corresponding thigh. Following the language outlined in Chapter 11 on hypnotherapy, the progressive relaxation from the forehead should be started with particular emphasis of relaxation on the cheeks, lips, and mouth area. In the event the dental assistant has conducted the progressive relaxation technique, the dentist should continue with the remaining relaxation procedure unless the patient has exhibited good rapport with the assistant.

The language between patient and hypnotist (dentist or dental assistant) should continue somewhat as follows:

I'm sure you realize that, even though you are somewhat relaxed, you can relax even more than you are now experiencing. And since the more relaxed you are, the less sensitive your nerve endings are. Why don't we get you to relax so much that you completely eliminate any feeling in those bothersome nerves?

I'm going to count back from ten and with each decreasing number, your body does relax even deeper and deeper. Each decreasing number causes your muscles to let go and relax. I want you to expect, feel, and cooperate in relaxing the muscles as we proceed ...

Ten ... now let your shoulders relax ... let them completely relax ... allow each and every large and small muscle to let go and relax ...

Nine ... send that relaxation down your right arm ... all the way through each muscle from your shoulder down to your elbow ... and now continuing down to your wrist ... allow those muscles to relax and let go ... now that relaxation continues down through the palms of your hands ... into your fingers and right to the ends of those fingers ... let that arm just lie there ...

Eight ...
(Follow the same procedure with the left arm.)

Seven ... allow that relaxation to flow down from your hands into the thighs ... let that feeling of comfort enter those thigh muscles ...

Six ... send the relaxation down the right leg, and allow each of your thigh muscles to grow pleasantly relaxed ...

Five ... just let those muscles feel relaxed and comfortable ... all the way down to your knees ... enjoy that feeling of comfort ...

Four ... now that feeling of relaxation continues down your right leg through each muscle down to the ankle, <u>causing</u> each muscle to let go and relax ... let that relaxation pass on down into your foot and into your toes ... feel that whole right leg relaxing and growing numb with relaxation.

Three ... now that feeling of relaxation continues to flow from your left hand down into your thigh muscles of your left leg ... just let it progress downward, <u>causing</u> those thigh muscles to relax ...

Two ... let that relaxation now continue down from your knee all the way into the ankle ... feel each muscle relaxing ... let them relax . . .

And one ... let that feeling of comfort flow down into your foot and into your toes, <u>causing</u> the whole leg to just let go and relax.

The preceding relaxation may be conducted either by the dentist or his assistant, depending upon the relationship of the patient to the dentist. However, the following verbiage should be carried out by the dentist as it gives the patient the feeling that he is now ready for and deserving of the attention of the dentist:

I'm going to slide my hand under your right hand and now with our palms touching, I want you to press against me until I tell you to LET GO, at which time you will release the pressure and <u>cause</u> your whole arm to become deeply and totally relaxed. Now press against my hand ... let go.

(Repeat this as often as necessary until the arm becomes absolutely limp, at which time you may then proceed to relax the left arm in a similar fashion.)

Now, I am going to gently rub the back of your right hand, and as I do so it <u>causes</u> the hand to become numb and useless ... and maybe even cold ... all the feeling in that hand from the wrist to the end of your fingers growing more numb and useless ... and now all the feeling of sensation and touch leaving ... disappearing ... going ... going ... and gone.

I am now going to raise the right hand up ... up to your jaw and as your hand touches the jaw, it <u>causes</u> the jaw muscles and nerves to become numb and useless ... all that feeling from your useless hand being absorbed into the jaw muscles and nerves, <u>causing</u> muscles and nerves to become absolutely and totally numb and useless ... let this feeling gently flow from your hand into your jaw, <u>causing</u> the whole area to grow numb and as that feeling flows from your hand into the jaw, each cell, nerve, and muscle becomes progressively more numb ... now I am going to gently separate your lips and rub your gums, <u>causing</u> the numbness to concentrate in the area that I rub ... feel the gum area growing totally and absolutely numb ... progressively more and more numb as I continue to rub this area ... now totally and completely numb.

Each and every time I place my hands on your shoulders like this ...

(Place your hands on the patient's shoulders.)

... and gently push like this ... (Push.) ... I am suggesting relaxation and whenever I do this, it <u>causes</u>

your eyes to become tired and your eyelids heavy with
relaxation ... and as I continue to exert a little pressure,
it <u>causes</u> your eyelids to close and <u>causes</u> you to go deep
into relaxation ... and you will relax just as deep as you
are now ... your arms and legs completely relaxed ...
and as your eyelids close, it <u>causes</u> your mouth muscles
to relax and <u>causes</u> your gums to become totally and
completely numb ... and as I gently rub your jaw like
this ...

(Gently rub the patient's jaw.)

... it <u>causes</u> the gums to become progressively more
numb and useless ... and now growing more numb ...
very numb ... totally numb.

The preceding paragraph constitutes a posthypnotic
suggestion, permitting a fast induction on future visits. The
hypnotist should select one or two methods of creating instant
inductions for subsequent visits, and these methods employed
should be noted on the patient's chart to eliminate embarrassment
should the patient fail to respond to any other method.

Chemical anesthesia may be used when the patient has not
satisfactorily responded to the suggestions of complete and total
numbness in the jaw and gum area. At this point, the patient should
be sufficiently relaxed so that no apprehension should be
experienced during such injection.

While performing dental work on the patient, it may be
noted that there could be a tendency for the patient to deepen and
lighten the hypnotic state. To alleviate this, it should be explained
to the patient that at any time he desires to more fully relax, all he
needs to do is raise and lower his right index finger in a pumping
fashion, causing his body to proceed to relax to any depth that he
may desire. This suggestion puts him in charge of his depth,

removing any fears that he may accidentally awaken or become fully aware, thereby experiencing unnecessary pain. Additionally, this will clue in the dentist as to the depth and condition of his patient.

CHILD INDUCTION TECHNIQUE

Draw a picture of a face on the thumbnail of the child, explaining to the child that you are drawing a face and "these are the eyes, nose, mouth, hair," etc. The drawing should be very slow and deliberate, done while directing the child's attention to every movement of the pen or pencil being used. When the picture has been completed, you may start speaking as follows:

I want you to look at, concentrate on, and stare at

the picture that we just drew on the back of your

thumbnail ... And soon the picture will cause your eyes

to become moist and watery, and make you feel drowsy

and sleepy.

(Now slowly, very slowly, move the thumb closer and closer to the bridge of the nose, continuing to speak in a mild and slow manner.)

Look at this picture and feel how it is making you

drowsy and sleepy ... your eyes becoming moist and

eyes starting to close to make them feel better. Now

your eyes are very tired and you are getting very drowsy

and soon your eyes will close and you will relax and

become sleepy ... now your eyes are closed, and you are

relaxing and beginning to go deep asleep ... let those

eyes remain closed and sleep.

This is the only induction where it is recommended that the terminology of "eyes closed" and "sleep" be used. Children associate sleeping with having the eyes closed while adults close the "eyelids" and associate sleep with being in a state of unconsciousness or being unaware.

ADDIITONAL FACTORS

The eye fixation method of induction may be utilized in a various number of ways. Group induction may be obtained by having the selected subjects fix their gaze upon a lit candle placed on the top step of a six-foot ladder. It must be remembered that anyone present during group demonstrations who can observe the object of concentration and can hear the language of the hypnotist, is a candidate for hypnosis. So whenever conducting a group hypnosis, look around to see if anyone else may have entered into a state of hypnosis.

An assistant or nurse can play an important part in relieving the subject's tension and apprehension prior to the induction procedure. The nurse or assistant is usually the medium of communication between the subject and the hypnotist from the initial visits through the last session. The acceptance of this role removes most of the apprehension on the part of the patient to any induction technique that may be employed later, and this is especially true in the treatment of children. Simple prearranged suggestions that the session will produce relaxation, comfort, and cure play an important part in the success of the sessions.

Once the subject is comfortably seated or lying down (as the case may be), the assistant or nurse may proceed in a casual manner, saying something like this:

> Why don't you make yourself comfortable and uncross your legs? Let your arms hang loosely along your sides and just close your eyes. In a moment, I am going to count from one to five and then back from five to one, and while I am counting from one to five I want

you to slowly take in a deep breath, and then slowly
exhale as I count backward from five to one. Now slowly
breathe in ... one ... two ... three ... four... and five.
Now exhale slowly ... five ... four ... three ... two ...
and one. Why don't we do it again?

(Repeat the process two more times by which time the subject
should be mildly exhausted.)

Now concentrate on relaxing your muscles and
getting just as comfortable as you can and (use name of
hypnotist) will be right in.

The assistant's or nurse's help may be utilized in setting
the pattern for posthypnotic suggestions or reinduction. As soon as
the subject has entered into a light state of hypnosis, posthypnotic
suggestion for reinduction should be given. Any simple suggestion
is sufficient, for example:

Whenever I or (name of hypnotist) asks you to
close your eyes and count from one to five as you take a
deep breath, you experience a feeling of comfort and
relaxation. And as you release the air counting backward
from five to one, you do go deeper and deeper into a
state of pleasant relaxation, feeling more and more
comfortable and relaxed. Each and every time that you
exhale, it causes you to relax even deeper and deeper.

Posthypnotic suggestions for reinduction should always be
administered immediately after the subject has entered into a light
state of hypnosis and restated at intervals during the hypnotic
sessions for emphasis. Since all suggestions may be accepted or
rejected by the subject, they must be phrased in such a manner that
their acceptance is assured. For many years, I have used the
following three posthypnotic suggestions without any active or
passive rejection:

(1)

Each and every time that I suggest relaxation, you do relax pleasantly and deeply.

(2)

Whenever I suggest relaxation, it causes your eyes to become tired and your eyelids do become heavy with relaxation and your eyelids close and you do relax pleasantly and deeply.

(3)

Each and every subsequent time that you relax, you relax more quickly and more deeply than the previous time. In other words, whenever you relax, you relax deeper than the time before.

These suggestions are given immediately *after* the induction technique has been completed and *before* the deepening processes have been commenced, and in the order listed. During the progressive relaxation, these suggestions should be repeated several times.

At this time, the subject usually is not aware that he has been hypnotized, as he is not experiencing a change in awareness and is fully cognizant of his surrounding circumstances and conditions. Not recognizing that a change from the conscious awareness to the subconscious awareness has taken place, the subject doesn't realize that each and every suggestion made by the hypnotist is accepted unless actively rejected. Once the suggestion is made and passively accepted by the subject, all that remains is to enhance the acceptability by compounding the suggestion. Repetition leads to increased acceptance and usually instant induction.

The first posthypnotic suggestion stating "each and every time that I suggest relaxation to you, you do relax pleasantly and deeply" is the most important and should be repeated at regular intervals during the deepening processes and therapy. Just slide in the suggestion between any sentences at any time. Any one of the other two suggestions may accompany the first suggestion or may be repeated several times as a separate suggestion. Repetition of the suggestion is the important thing as this causes those suggestions to become buried deep in the memory bank, resulting in a positive and immediate response.

I prefer to call the first suggestion the "umbrella clause" since it may be implemented by any number of the following applications:

(1)

By placing my hand in this position, I am suggesting relaxation. And each and every time that I suggest relaxation, you do relax pleasantly and deeply. And it causes your eyes to become tired and your eyelids to grow so heavy with relaxation that they do close, and you do relax pleasantly and deeply.

(2)

By brushing my hair with my hand like this, I am suggesting relaxation and ...
(Complete the sentence as above.)

(3)

By rubbing my nose with my handkerchief like this, I am suggesting relaxation and ... (etc.)

(4)

By crossing my legs like this, I am suggesting relaxation and ... (etc.)

(5)

By rubbing my ear with my fingers like this, I am suggesting relaxation and ... (etc.)

(6)

Whenever I pick up a pencil (or glass of water,
book, this paper, pencil, or any other selected object),
I am suggesting relaxation and ... (etc.)

(7)

The suggestion of relaxation and reinduction may be
implemented by any means or method that the hypnotist may
select by simply stating: As I do this ... (name whatever you
select), I am suggesting relaxation and ... (etc.)

Since every patient or subject will return for more than the
initial session, such reinduction at subsequent sessions can be
utilized in a matter of seconds. However, reinduction is most
effective when rehearsed during the initial session at a time when
the hypnotist is satisfied after testing that at least a deep state of
hypnosis has been attained. The rehearsal of the reinduction
technique during the initial session will usually cause the patient
or subject to enter into a deeper state of hypnosis, making the person
more responsive to the posthypnotic suggestions. The visual
observation permits the subject to become thoroughly familiar with
the reinduction technique so that reinduction may occur without
any verbal suggestions. In most cases, when the subject observes
the hypnotist going through the suggested motions, reinduction
will be spontaneous.

The posthypnotic suggestions for reinduction should be
given after the initial induction, deepening processes, and therapy
have been completed. Reinduction suggestion may be given as
follows:

Each and every time I suggest relaxation to you, you
do relax pleasantly and deeply. Now still remaining
deeply relaxed, I want you to open your eyes and look at
the palm of my hand. By placing my hand in this

position, I am suggesting relaxation and each time I

suggest relaxation, your eyelids grow tired. And your

eyelids feel heavy and cause your eyelids to close. And

as I lower my hand closer to your forehead, this causes

your eyes to become progressively more tired and your

eyelids heavy with relaxation and your eyelids do close.

(Now lower your hands, causing the eyelids to close and reinducting the subject.)

With the initial induction, deepening processes, and therapy completed; and before the end of the session, while the subject is still in a state of hypnosis, another reinduction technique may be introduced as follows:

Each and every time I suggest relaxation, you do

relax pleasantly and deeply. <u>Still remaining deeply</u>

<u>relaxed</u>, open your eyes and look at me.

(Hypnotist gently brushes his hair with the palm of his hand.)

By brushing my hair with the palm of my hand, I am

suggesting relaxation and whenever I suggest relaxation,

it causes your eyes to become tired and your eyelids to

become heavy and causes your eyelids to close.

(Continue brushing the hair.)

Experience your eyes becoming progressively more

and more tired and your eyelids growing heavier and

heavier and closing ... relaxing and closing ... closing

and closed.

When the subject has become familiar with the reinduction technique, then at subsequent sessions the subject is asked to sit in the chair and get into a comfortable position. At this time, the hypnotist may proceed as follows:

I want you to notice that I am brushing my hair with
the palm of my hand and I told you at our last session
that whenever I do this, I am suggesting relaxation. So
keep looking as I brush my hair with my palm and
experience how it causes your eyes to become tired and
your eyelids to grow heavy with relaxation, progressively
more relaxed as I continue to brush my hair. Now eyelids
are growing progressively heavier and heavier and
closing and closing ... closing ... and closed.

The enactment and reenactment of posthypnotic suggestions for induction at subsequent sessions result in an automatic
induction and also serve another purpose in convincing the subject
that he has been hypnotized. At the conclusion of the initial session,
over 90 percent of the subjects will deny, some with reservations,
that they had ever been hypnotized. Therefore. I like to conduct a
challenge with the subject – not a challenge between the hypnotist
and the subject, but a challenge between the subject's conscious
and subconscious mind.

With the subject still in a state of hypnosis, the challenge
goes something like this:

You will remember earlier that I stated to you that
each and every time I suggest relaxation, you do relax
pleasantly and deeply and the suggestion causes your
eyes to become tired and your eyelids heavy and they do
close?

(The subject answers "yes.")

At that time, I was talking to your subconscious
mind and you also remember that during our
conversation earlier I explained to you that you were not
able to overcome that drive started by your

subconscious mind and that the subconscious mind was
more powerful than your conscious mind and that was
the reason you couldn't change and stop doing the
things that you know caused you harm, such as smoking
cigarettes?

(The subject answers "yes.")

Now you are going to learn that when there is a
conflict between the conscious desire and the
subconscious desire, the subconscious does always
prevail and win. Still remaining deeply relaxed, I want
you to open your eyes. I am going to place my hand
over your head and I want you to look at the palm of my
hand.

(Place hand in position.)

I have instructed your subconscious mind that when
I do this, it causes your eyes to become tired and your
eyelids to grow heavy and they do close before my hand
touches your forehead. I want you to use all your
conscious effort and try to keep your eyelids open. Try
as hard as you can, but you will find that the eyelids do
close, whether you like it or not.

(Now start to lower the hand very slowly.)

You can feel your eyes growing tired and your
eyelids growing heavy with relaxation and beginning to
close. Eyelids very heavy, so heavy that you can't keep
them up. Feel your eyelids relaxing and closing ...
closing ... closing and closed. Why, your eyelids closed
before my hand even touched your forehead.

Still remaining deeply relaxed, I want you to open your eyelids and let's do it again. But this time, try harder than the last time and you will find that the harder you try, the quicker your eyelids do close. Once again, look at the palm of my hand ...
(Place your hand over the forehead.)

... and this time, I am not going to say one word to you. I will just lower my hand and before my hand touches your forehead, your eyelids will be closed.
(Slowly lower hand.)

Now they are closed, closed so tightly, you cannot open them and the harder you try, the tighter they stick together, so tight, they do not open. Try to open your eyes and you do find that they do not open ...

Stop trying. They won't open. Maybe now you can more fully understand something about hypnosis and your subconscious mind. When your subconscious mind receives a suggestion or instruction, either intentionally or unintentionally, and when that instruction or suggestion becomes buried deep within, there is very little your conscious effort can do to overcome its effect. Your conscious mind cannot penetrate the necessary depth to erase that suggestion. It is necessary through the process of hypnosis to descend to the proper depth of your subconscious mind and remove the problem suggestion and restore some sense of normalcy to your behavior patterns. You see, you didn't have much choice controlling your problems from the beginning. So why

don't we get on with the business of getting rid of those
unwanted deep-seated problems? ...

At the count of three, your eyes do open and you do
feel perfectly wonderful in mind and body. One ... two
... and three. Open your eyes, feeling fine.

Without ever discussing it, you have restored in the subject
his self-confidence. For months and maybe years, he has quietly
but persistently condemned himself for not having the willpower
and self-confidence to be able to control his conduct in the manner
he knows to be the most beneficial. He has been given an "out" by
your explanation and suggestion that the problem was so deep-
seated, the conscious mind couldn't penetrate the necessary depth
to give him some relief. Hypnosis becomes more logical and
acceptable. A possible cure for his problems becomes more of a
reality which, in turn, leads to a cure.

8

DEEPENING PROCESSES

Hypnosis is a very easy phenomenon to bring about. The technique is so simple in principle, any talented person can hypnotize a cooperative subject. When hypnosis is understood, we realize that each of us continually enters into a state of hypnosis a minimum of one hundred times each and every day. Memory recall, such as thinking about yesterday's activities, is a light form of hypnosis as are mental calculations of mathematics. Whenever a person utilizes information deposited in the memory bank, hypnosis is created.

As explained earlier in this book, hypnosis is a state of awareness dominated by the subconscious mind – that is, that portion of the mind that uses the information deposited at some earlier time in the memory bank. Whenever a person "thinks," he enters into a very light state of hypnosis. Other than bringing forth some information that lies on the edge or perimeter of the memory bank, light hypnosis has very little, if any, therapeutic value. In this state, there is very little relaxation. The subject can waiver in and out of hypnosis with relative ease and without being aware of his actions.

In order to be productive and bring about the necessary desired results, the subject must be permitted to enter a deeper state. Many of the so-called "authorities on hypnosis" describe in publications and books that, based on their experiences, only about one-fourth of their subjects are able to enter into a deep state of hypnosis and approximately one-tenth are able to enter the deepest somnambulistic state. Such statements support my position that these "authorities" fail to understand hypnosis and lack the knowledge and ability to obtain the deepest state. My experiences and that of my students show that approximately 95 percent of cooperative subjects are able to enter into a somnambulistic state within the first two sessions.

Several organizations and societies that advance and promote hypnosis have attempted to standardize or classify the various levels of the states of hypnosis without success. A light state of hypnosis is accomplished by merely closing the eyelids. As explained earlier, closing of the eyelids shuts down one-eighth of the conscious awareness. In each eye, there are 120 million cells called rods and cones. These cells are sensitive to light, movement, and color. Closing of the eyelids shuts down 240 million cells. In addition, 30 thousand to 50 thousand optic nerves that convey information from the eyes to the visual cortex are closed down. Hundreds of thousands of nerves that correlate vision and physical movement are shut down. The eyes are "windows to the brain" and with closing the windows, the conscious awareness is diminished by one-eighth. As the conscious awareness is diminished, the subconscious awareness is elevated one-eighth. And so it now becomes necessary to diminish the conscious awareness further by utilizing deepening techniques.

Although some authorities recommend testing at this stage by eye and limb catalepsy, I am strongly opposed to it. Any negative result – for example, when the hypnotist suggests that the subject cannot open his eyelids yet the eyelids pop open – creates increased apprehension and doubt. It is difficult enough to convince the subject that he has been hypnotized without creating additional problems. I strongly recommend that no testing be done on any subject, no matter what his appearance may be, until the progressive relaxation and one additional deepening process have been completed. As long as it is necessary to conduct these deepening processes, I see no need for any prior testing.

When the progressive relaxation process has been done in a low, calculated, and deliberate manner, the subject should be in a medium state of hypnosis. However, I have found that in many cases, if the progressive relaxation is properly utilized, a subject can enter into a deep state. In any event, I recommend that at least two deepening techniques be administered before any testing is done. Should the number method be used, it is important to remember the last number that is audibly spoken by the subject. When counting backward from one hundred, the last audible number is an indication of the depth of the subject. Ceasing to count before ninety-five is reached indicates that the subject is in a deep state of hypnosis, between ninety-five and eighty-five indicates a light state, and anything after eighty should alert the hypnotist that the subject is in a light state of hypnosis and very likely a difficult and non-cooperative subject. At the commencement of the backward count, the numbers will be very audible, and with each decreasing number, there should be less movement of the lips until there is a mere whisper.

PROGRESSIVE RELAXATION

Progressive relaxation is the process whereby the subject is directed to concentrate on relaxing each and every muscle and area of the body from the forehead down to the toes. The hypnotist directs the attention of the subject to various areas of the body and by his concentration, he causes those muscles and areas of the body to relax. This is a subject-oriented exercise in relaxation and when it is mastered by the subject under the direction of the hypnotist, self-hypnosis is the result. (In Chapter 11 on hypnotherapy, this procedure is outlined in detail.) Terminology enhances the subject's concentration and participation, thereby eliminating outside stimuli and interference. Terminology such as the following are some examples:

(1)

Send the relaxation down to ...

(2)

Let the relaxation flow from your (...) to your (...)

(3)

Experience those muscles relaxing ...

(4)

Think about relaxing your (...)

Concentration and focusing of the attention bring about subtle induction and depth of hypnosis in resistant persons.

Progressive relaxation may be employed to hypnotize anxious, apprehensive, and resistant persons by asking them to adjust themselves to a comfortable position and close their eyelids. When this has been accomplished, the hypnotist says:

I am going to teach you the progressive relaxation

method so that any time you so desire, you will be able

to relax your entire body and remove all the tension so

you can enjoy the daily activities.

Start slowly, permitting the subject to follow your directions, leaving ample time for him to create the feeling of relaxation in the various areas. With the proper timing and sequence, relaxation should have settled into the entire body by the time the area of the toes has been reached, with the subject in a light or medium state of hypnosis without his being aware of what has happened. Since the subject is totally aware and cognizant of his surroundings and since it appears to him that nothing has been done to hypnotize him, he will refuse to admit that he has been hypnotized unless there is some manifestation of an observed technique.

COUNTING BACKWARD

This is by far the most common and widely used method of developing a deeper state of hypnosis within the subject. (Since this technique will be explained thoroughly in Chapter 11 on hypnotherapy, it serves no purpose to explain it in detail in this chapter.)

Count backward to deepen the relaxation and forward for awakening purposes. Be consistent. I prefer to commence with the number one hundred as this allows adequate room to continue the counting process, whereas starting with a much lower number, such as twenty, leaves little time to develop relaxation in a resistant person. Since this resistance is not already noticeable, this might lead to the appearance of failure. Once the induction and deepening process have been successful, counting backward from ten may be adequate for self-hypnosis.

ALPHABET

The alphabet deepening process, in my opinion, is the best deepening technique ever developed. This deepening technique combines two methods: (1) each movement of the eraser causes the subject to relax more and more and (2) by the addition of stress, his conscious mind decides to stop. While the subject is writing and erasing the letters of the alphabet, the hypnotist is talking about other letters of the alphabet which, in turn, causes stress in the subject. The subject is trying to concentrate on one letter and at the same time hearing other letters of the alphabet. This is the conscious mind trying to follow what is going on. Finally, the conscious mind decides to stop following both of these activities. At that time, the subject is unaware that he has entered into a deeper state of hypnosis. (This alphabet technique is also detailed in Chapter 11 on hypnotherapy.) Master this technique, and success ratio is quicker and lasts longer.

The classroom is where you begin to create imagery in the subject. The more often certain words are repeated, the more distinct the image is created. You will notice in the chapter on hypnotherapy how often certain words are repeated.

USING THE STAIRWAY

Picture or imagine yourself standing at the top of a stairway.

You look down and see these steps as they descend downward, downward. If you like, the stairs can go straight down, or they can go to a landing and turn and descend to another landing, then continue down to the different landings, whichever you like.

So have in mind that you're standing at the top of the stairway looking down the steps. And there is a handrail next to the stairs. As you stand at the top of the stairway, place one hand on the handrail and then slowly start walking down the steps, taking one step down and then another.

Each and every step you take causes you to go deeper and deeper into relaxation. Continue your steps downward, downward and deeper, and every step you take causes you to relax even deeper and deeper.

Walk down toward the basement of your relaxation, always feeling more comfortable, more pleasant with each and every step that you take. So let the stairway take you down, pleasantly walking and going deeper and deeper.

Your hand on the handrail guides you as you descend deeper and deeper, and as you continue to step downward, downward, you do find that your legs are becoming weaker and weaker, hardly able to step downward as your body relaxes more and more, stepping down and going deeper and deeper. Every step you take causes you to go deep, deep into relaxation, feeling more comfortable, more pleasant, and more relaxed.

Nothing bothers you. Nothing disturbs you. Should you hear anything other than my voice, all it does is cause you to relax even deeper and deeper, more pleasant, peaceful in mind and body.

Continue to slowly step down, down, down. When you have reached the last step, you will notice there is a closed door at the bottom of this landing. So once you have reached the bottom of the stairway, look around and when you see the closed door at the bottom of the stairway, nod your head YES so that I know you have seen the closed door.

(The subject nods his head "yes.")

Behind the door is a library. You know what a library looks like: many, many bookshelves, bookshelves in so many, many rows. And on these bookshelves are so very many, many books. Go over to the library door, open the library door, step into the library, and close the library door behind you.

(Continue thereafter with the library activities as outlined also in Chapter 11 on hypnotherapy.)

In the event that the therapist has the subject in the classroom and the alphabet deepening process is not sufficient to have the person in a relative deep state of hypnosis, then insert the stairway deepening before the subject enters into the library. Use the following language:

Look around in the classroom and when you see a closed door, nod your head YES.

(The subject nods his head "yes.")

The door you are now looking at leads to a hallway.
In the hallway is a stairway. So go over to the hallway
door, open the hallway door, step into the hallway, and
close the hallway door behind you. Now look around in
this hallway and when you see the stairway, walk over to
the stairway and stand at the top of the stairway.

This way you can get the patient from the classroom to the
stairway instead of having the patient picture and imagine that he
is standing at the top of the stairway. When the patient is at the top
of the stairway, then the therapist may continue as set in the
beginning of this stairway deepening process.

Using Falling Leaves

I want you to imagine or picture that you are lying on
a very nice grassy spot – someone's lawn, a grassy
meadow, or some place you may have been before, or just
picture lying on this beautiful green grass and looking up
at the blue daylight sky. Feel the warm breeze on your
face and body ... and everything is quiet and peaceful.

Close by is a tree ... a big, tall, tree and as the
breeze is gently blowing, you hear the rustling of the
leaves and everything else is quiet, pleasant, and
relaxing.

As you continue to look straight up into the sky, you
may even see some birds with their wings spread, gently
gliding with the wind. You may even notice some white
clouds slowly drifting by, so peaceful, quiet, relaxing,
comfortable, pleasant, serene, and enjoyable. And as you

slowly glance over to the tree, you see the leaves quietly moving with the wind. And now one of the leaves comes loose and gently floats down, down ever so slowly, drifting down toward you. And as that leaf comes down, falling, falling, it causes you to go deeper and deeper into relaxation. The gently falling leaf, coming down so quietly and so peacefully, causes you to relax even deeper and deeper and deeper.

Now the leaf slowly settles to the ground, relaxing you pleasantly and comfortably.

As you look back at the top of the tree, another leaf separates from the branch and starts drifting down, causing you to go even deeper and deeper into relaxation, feeling more comfortable and more pleasant, deeply relaxing. And as you continue to see the leaf coming down, way in the distant sky, the white clouds are drifting by, peaceful and quiet. And the leaf still keeps coming down, down, slowly coming down and gently settling on the ground, causing you to go deeper and deeper into relaxation, feeling more comfortable and pleasant and totally relaxed.

So let yourself go, close your eyes, and let go and relax, relax.

With this technique, the therapist can use as many leaves that may be necessary to get the subject into a deep state of hypnosis. It is always important to continuously observe the subject during the session for any physical movements that may give the impression that the subject feels uneasy. This you will notice by any movement of the hands or feet.

OPENING AND CLOSING OF EYES

As you sit in that comfortable chair, in a moment I will ask you to open your eyes and then slowly close them. And each and every time you close your eyes, this causes you to relax even deeper and deeper, always doubling your relaxation with each movement of the eyelids as they close.

Now very carefully and slowly, open your eyes. That's fine.

Now very slowly and carefully, close them. And let the eyelids come down ever so slowly, sending you deeper and deeper and deeper into relaxation and very relaxed. Let the relaxation flow from your eyelids down through your cheeks and down to your shoulders and down into your body.

Now once again slowly, open the eyelids and very carefully and very slowly, close the eyelids just as slowly as you possibly can. Gently close the eyelids and let that relaxation flow down through your body, causing you to go deeper and deeper into relaxation, drifting ever so deep and so relaxed. As your eyelids close, this causes your eyelids to grow heavy, heavy eyelids, and heavy with relaxation. You hardly can open them, but let's do it again.

Slowly open the eyes. That's fine. Now once again, let your eyelids close by themselves. Your eyelids are growing heavier and heavier, closing and relaxing deeper and deeper. Close the eyelids and let the relaxation go through your whole body. Just let go and relax, relax.

This technique of opening and closing the eyelids can continue until the therapist is satisfied that the subject has difficulty trying to lift the eyelids.

PLACING HAND ON FOREHEAD

I am gently going to place my hand on your forehead, and you do feel the touch. Feel my fingers on your forehead.

Feel the point of touch growing warm, pleasantly warm, the warmth of my fingers seeping into your forehead and gently flowing down into your body from the forehead down, down to the neck, continuing down to the shoulders and through your body. Accept this warm feeling of comfort and relaxation.

So let this warmth flow down, touching every muscle, causing every muscle to relax and let go. Feel the warmth as it comes down, down through your cheeks and down into the neck, and let it flow across your shoulders and down your arms to your fingertips. Let the warmth relax you and bring about a warm, pleasant, comfortable feeling that flows from your shoulders down through your chest and down your back, down into your stomach and settling down into the hips, relaxing every muscle, every nerve, every cell, and every fiber as it slowly goes downward, downward and deeper and deeper and deeper into a feeling of relaxation.

Accept this feeling of relaxation and let it flow, and now as this relaxation continues to flow down from your hips down through both of your legs, relax every muscle in both of your legs. Every large and small muscle all the way down to the knees and continuing past the knees down through the muscles, down to the ankles, and into the feet and right to your toes. So let those legs grow limp and relaxed. Let those arms relax, and make your body relax. The warmth relaxes your body, sending you deeper and deeper.

Nothing bothers you and nothing disturbs you. Should you hear anything other than my voice, all it can do is cause you to go deeper and deeper into relaxation, always feeling more comfortable and more pleasant and more relaxed. So let yourself drift deeper and deeper and deeper. Just let go and enjoy that feeling of complete and total relaxation, always drifting deeper and deeper.

RAISING AND LOWERING THE ARM

I am going to lift your arm ...

(The right or left arm may be used.)

... by grasping the wrist and gently lifting the arm. Let me lift your arm. Don't you exercise any movement of any muscle. No effort, please.

I am going to place my other hand on your shoulder gently. And I am going to lift your arm up and extend your arm, gently and easily, straight out from your shoulder.

(Extend the subject's arm.)

And now as I lower the arm, it causes you to relax even deeper and deeper. The movement of the arm, as it is lowered, causes your whole body to let go and relax. So let yourself relax, relax. As the arm is further lowered, it causes you to relax even deeper, deeply relaxing and relaxing.

(About four inches before the arm comes to rest, gently let the arm drop so that it falls limply into position. If you are not satisfied that complete relaxation has been obtained, proceed with the same deepening process with the other arm.)

DEEPENING TECHNIQUE WITH PASSING OF TIME

As you continue to sit in that chair, each passing moment causes you to relax even deeper and deeper and feel, as you continue to sit in that chair, your body is relaxing, more pleasant, more comfortable, more relaxed, always drifting deeper and deeper – let nothing bother you, nothing disturb you. Continue to relax even deeper and deeper with each passing moment, and each breath you take causes you to drift deeper and deeper. So just sit there and relax.

I want you to take in one deep breath and hold it ... hold it ... and now slowly exhale, causing you to drift deeper and deeper as you exhale.

So why don't you exhale all tension out of your body and let each passing moment send you deeper and deeper into relaxation? So do it once again.

Take a deep breath very slowly and carefully – a little bit more and hold it ... hold it ... exhale, let it out slowly, very slowly, and let the passing moments relieve you of your tension ... so exhale your tension out and let go.

Relax and let the relaxation flow from the top of your head all the way down through your body right down to your toes and your fingertips. Just let go ... let go. All you have to do for the rest of the session is sit there in that chair and just relax and let me do the work. As the session continues, each passing moment causes you to relax even deeper and deeper ... so let go and relax ... relax.

These deepening techniques are just a few of the varied methods used by hypnotists. Every hypnotist has a tendency to change or modify any one or more methods, depending upon his own particular style or degree of success. Whatever method used or created in deepening the state of hypnosis, the application of cause and effect should be employed. Whenever the subject concentrates, thinks, or imagines that something is happening, that thought process causes the subject to relax and as that event is happening, the relaxation is taking place. In other words, the relaxation takes place concurrently with the thought of the event in the mind of the subject.

At the time of interviewing the subject, his hobbies should be discussed, giving rise to developing a deepening process. Suppose the subject enjoys fishing. Then he should imagine he is on a boat, drifting close to the shore and as he slowly passes each tree along the shoreline, it causes him to drift deeper and deeper into relaxation and with each passing tree, he is going deeper and deeper, feeling more comfortable and more relaxed. Every cast of the fishing line causes him to go deeper into relaxation or every turn of the reel causes him to drift deeper and deeper into relaxation.

There are no limits to the techniques a hypnotist may develop for use in deepening the state of hypnosis. As long as the word "causes" is used, any number of events can be utilized as a deepening technique.

Here are several examples:

(1)

As you listen to my voice, each word that you hear causes you to relax deeper and deeper.

(2)

As you listen to the music, each beat causes you to relax progressively more and more.

(3)

As you hear the air-conditioner, this causes you to relax progressively more and more.

(4)

As you hear the traffic outside, this causes you to relax more and more.

(5)

As you smell the aroma, this causes you to relax deeper and deeper.

(6)

As you feel the texture of the material on the recliner that you are on, this causes you to relax even deeper and deeper.

9

TESTS OF DEPTH OF HYPNOSIS

In all phases of hypnosis, it is the subject's thought that creates the condition and body responses; therefore it should be obvious that the success or failure of the test is directly related to the manner in which the suggestion is framed. There are several reasons for conducting the tests during the hypnotic session, the main being to apprise the hypnotist of the depth of the subject prior to the commencement of the suggestive therapy.

When one is conducting sessions for behavioral changes, no tests should be conducted until after the progressive relaxation and at least one deepening process have been conducted. Premature testing might result in a negative response, thereby heightening the apprehension of the subject and creating doubt in his mind as to his state of hypnosis. Every negative response to any test raises the level of the depth of hypnosis, and every doubt created has a tendency to cause rejection of subsequent suggestions, especially those related to further testing of depth.

When there is a positive response to the test conducted, confidence in hypnosis is increased, bringing about further expectations of successful treatment.

Recognition by the subject of his inability to perform certain simple physical movements convinces the subject that he has indeed been hypnotized. Once this recognition has been established within the mind of the subject, acceptance of the suggestive therapy follows as a matter of course, resulting in an automatic deepening of the hypnotic state, removing any residue of passive resistance. The implementation of the posthypnotic suggestion for reinduction causes the subject to enter a deep state of hypnosis in a matter of seconds during all subsequent visits.

Proper testing is an important element to be considered, especially during the first hypnotic session.

Several organizations and societies that advance and promote hypnosis have attempted to standardize or classify the various levels of the states of hypnosis without much success. These levels of hypnosis may be classified as:

- Light
- Mild
- Medium
- Deep
- Somnambulistic
- Esdaile

These classifications are so designated, depending upon the responses of the subjects to various tests conducted during the sessions. Some hypnotists will consider the light state of hypnosis as also being mild, whereas others would prefer to combine mild with medium, depending upon their successes with various subjects. There is a tendency for the depth to vary during each session and from session to session, so that where there has been obtained a positive result for a test for medium depth, a negative result might follow at the subsequent test. Intermittent testing should be conducted as the session progresses to maintain a level of responses, especially during the therapy part of the session.

Testing the subject to determine whether or not the subject has reached these respective depths takes practice, patience, and understanding. From the initial introduction and throughout the entire session, the hypnotist must be most observant of the anxiety and apprehension of the subject since there is a direct relationship between these and the depth that can be reached during the first session. Contrary to the opinion of most hypnotists, somnambulism can be obtained by most subjects when the proper methods and techniques are employed. The difficulty arises when shortcuts and hurried techniques are used for symptom removal before the subject is ready for this therapy.

When failure results, the hypnotist attributes this to the inability of the subject to reach the proper depth rather than his own inefficiencies. Every subject's response to the tests will vary, requiring personal observation of the subject while these tests are being conducted. Although the tapes on hypnosis may have some beneficial aspects for home use, they have no place in the hypnotist's office for use in induction, deepening, or therapy.

It is the response to most tests and not the test itself that will reveal to the hypnotist the depth of hypnosis within the subject. Notice what happens during the eye catalepsy test, after you have said to the subject: "Your eyelids are closed, so very tight that you cannot open them. The harder you try, the tighter they stick together … try to open them, but you will find that you cannot." Note the movement of the eye muscles and eyelids. Should the eyelids only flicker with some movement of the eyeballs, then the subject is in a light state of hypnosis. When there is no movement of the eyelids but some raising of the eyebrows, then the subject has reached the medium state. And when there is no movement of any eye muscles, then the subject is in a deep state of hypnosis.

The same is applied to the leg catalepsy. After the completion of the suggestions creating a numb and useless feeling in the leg, the hypnotist will state: "Now your leg is numb and useless, so useless you cannot lift it and cross it over the other leg. The harder you try, the more numb and useless your leg becomes, so that you are now unable to cross your legs. Try to cross your legs and you will find that you cannot." Should the leg be lifted and crossed without any difficulty, then the subject is in a light state of hypnosis.

In a light or mild state of hypnosis, the hypnotist should start with a test that requires very little physical activity. The usual tests for this light or mild state of hypnosis are the following:

- Catalepsy of the eyelids
- Catalepsy of the limbs

Should it appear during the testing that the eyelids are about to open after some fluttering or that the limbs can be easily moved, then the testing should be immediately stopped by merely saying, "Stop trying. That's all right. You don't have to try anymore." Go right into another deepening process without hesitation as the subject has not reached the necessary depth for therapeutic purposes. When the subject has reached the medium state of hypnosis, the following phenomena can be expected:

- Inhibition of voluntary movements
- Automatic obedience
- Limited induced personality changes
- Emotional changes
- Partial posthypnotic anesthesia
- Guidance therapy

When the subject has reached the deep state of hypnosis, the responses attributed to that depth may include:

- Expanded emotional changes
- Extensive anesthesia
- Age regression
- Automatic writing
- Simple posthypnotic suggestions
- Mild hallucinations
- Symptom removal by suggestions
- Desensitization

It should follow as a matter of course that when the hypnotist is satisfied with the responses of eye and limb catalepsy, then the more difficult tests should be conducted to determine the deep and somnambulistic states. Glove anesthesia and anesthesia transfer from one limb to another or from one part of the body to another part is appropriate. Testing the effectiveness of the anesthesia may be done with a pin or clamp with the subsequent responses indicating a deep or somnambulistic state of hypnosis.

The preferred state for symptom removal is somnambulism. When this state has been reached, there is an appearance of complete relaxation and non-responsiveness to suggestions for physical movement. For the uninformed, it would appear that the subject is sound asleep. The phenomena attributed to somnambulism are as follows:

- Ability to open the eyes without affecting the state of hypnosis
- Complete posthypnotic amnesia
- Positive and negative hallucinations
- Extreme posthypnotic suggestions
- Psychobiologic therapy (reconditioning)
- Drastic emotional changes
- Hypnoanalysis (regression and revivification)

The Esdaile state of hypnosis was named after Dr. James Esdaile, an English physician who practiced medicine in India and performed hundreds of major surgical procedures, using only hypnosis as an anesthetic. This also has been called "states below somnambulism." Contrary to popular opinion, this state of hypnosis may be achieved by most of the subjects when the proper deepening techniques are applied. This state is evidenced by a complete physical relaxation with no movement of the limbs upon suggestion and the inability to formulate audible vocal sounds properly. Although the subject can hear and recognize surrounding circumstances, there is the distinct lack of ability to make audible, responsive answers that can be understood easily. This state is primarily used in surgical procedures as the patient is usually totally anesthetized.

It must be emphasized that these various states of hypnosis must not be taken literally as some subjects may show different phenomena in certain states. Some patients in somnambulism may not follow posthypnotic suggestions while others in the medium or deep states will show traits of being in somnambulism. Since these exceptions occur frequently enough, constant monitoring by the hypnotist is required during each and every part of the sessions.

The two basic principles of hypnosis, need and belief, play an increasing role in developing and obtaining the necessary depth.

The capacity for somnambulism is within each of us; however, this capacity becomes limited by the lack of motivation and belief that hypnosis is the answer for symptomatic difficulties. Most of the psychobiologic therapies (such goals as guidance, education, and symptom removal) may be attained in the deep state of hypnosis. The state of somnambulism can have a more profound effect on the patient or subject than the earlier states. It is, therefore, important for the hypnotist to achieve as high a skill as possible in the induction and deepening techniques.

The tests used will largely depend upon the preference of the hypnotist and the success he has attained from its use. The eye and limb catalepsy tests usually are the first to be conducted by the hypnotist at the initial session; however, it must be understood that once one has enjoyed success with these tests, they should not be repeated again during that session.

The tests are for the sole purpose of determining the depth of the subject and not to be used in determining whether or not hypnosis has been effective. Although it has been disputed, I have always maintained and demonstrated that the subject enters into the primary or light state of hypnosis by merely closing the eyelids. The longer a subject remains in hypnosis and with each subsequent session, deeper states will be experienced. Guiding the subject to the necessary depth depends upon the ability and skills of the hypnotist and for this reason, detailed induction and deepening techniques have been presented in this book.

Remember, it is the response to the test and not the test itself that gives the hypnotist the needed information to establish the depth attained. When the subject is unable to lift the eyelids and open the eyes, a light state of hypnosis has been created; however, the same can be said about the deep or somnambulistic state. In such a deep state, the subject is also unable to lift the eyelids. To recognize the proper depth, the hypnotist must observe the subject's efforts in the performance of the tests. The more physical effort exhibited by the subject during the tests, the lighter the state of hypnosis and it follows that the less effort, the greater the depth.

EYE TEST (CATALEPSY)

Now your eyelids are closed and closed very tight. They're closed so tight you can't open them. They're glued together ... stuck together ... the harder you try to open them, the more difficult it is. Your eyelids are closed tight ... tight ... growing progressively tighter with each passing moment.

As you think about opening your eyelids, your thoughts cause your eyelids to grow progressively more limp and useless ... glued together ... stuck together ... even zipped together so that you cannot open your eyelids. So think about your eyelids and try to open your eyelids and you find your eyelids glued together ... stuck ... even zipped so that you cannot open the eyelids.

But go ahead and direct your attention to your eyelids and you find out that you cannot lift the eyelids. Try but you can't.

The success obtained in any testing is through the language that is used. Since every activity in the human body is the result of a thought, it is therefore the thought that causes the result. In every test in order to create an adverse result, there must be a thought that creates this result. In the language for the test, I say:

As you think about opening your eyelids, your thoughts cause your eyelids to become more limp, useless, glued together, stuck together so that you cannot open your eyelids.

Once your false statement becomes true, you know the person is in a state of hypnosis. The more physical effort required for the activity, the deeper the state of hypnosis needed.

Eye catalepsy can be achieved in a light state or in a deep state. This test will only reveal that a light state has been achieved. Subsequent more difficult tests will alert the hypnotist as to the depth of hypnosis.

RIGID ARM TEST

I'm going to hold your right arm by the wrist, and I will lift it straight up ... straight out ... put my other hand on your shoulder and as I squeeze your shoulder, it causes the shoulder muscles to become tight ... shoulder locked in place tight ... tight.

As I gently rub my hand from your shoulder to your elbow, the touch of my hand on each muscle causes every muscle to becomes stiff and rigid ... rigid ... rigid ... just as though your arm is turning into a steel bar ... so stiff and rigid nothing can move it. Nothing can bend it.

Now as I squeeze your elbow, it causes the elbow to lock tight ... tight ... so tight, it won' t bend ... and as I rub my hand from your elbow to your wrist, touching every muscle, causing every muscle to become stiff and rigid ... rigid ... your whole arm turning into a steel bar ... stiff and rigid ... nothing can move it and as I gently squeeze your wrist, the wrist locks into place tight ... tight ... your fingers are now extended, and every knuckle and muscle is locked in place tight ... tight ...

arms so rigid, so stiff ... you can't move it, can't bend it.

Still remaining deeply relaxed, I want you to open your eyes and look at your arm. I know you think you can move the arm but as you think about moving the arm or the fingers, your thoughts cause the arm to grow more stiff and rigid like a steel bar wrapped in steel bands ... so stiff and rigid, you can't move your arm. Try to move the arm but you find your arm totally stiff and rigid. Think about your arm and you try to move the arm. You can neither lower it nor lift it. Try to lift it. You will find it won't go up nor will it go down ... you cannot move it, cannot bend it ... locked in place tight ... tight.

As I gently rub your hand and your arm, it causes the muscles to release ... the joints to become unlocked and as I lower your hand, it causes your arm and hand to become perfectly normal in every respect. Now you can move it and as I continue lowering your arm, it causes the whole body to relax deeper and deeper.

OPEN HAND TEST

I want you to extend your right arm straight out from your chest and stretch your fingers out wide apart ... straight out and keep the fingers separated straight out ... straight out ... I'm going to count from five to one and each decreasing number causes your fingers to become stiffer and more rigid ... so stiff, you cannot bend them and can't close them.

Five ... fingers are getting stiff ... growing stiffer and stiffer.

Four ... fingers locked in place tight ... tight ... wrist locked in place tight.

Three ... fingers are extended ... every knuckle locked in place ... stiff and rigid ... stiff and rigid.

Two ... fingers are growing stiffer and more rigid ...

And one ... now so stiff and rigid, you can't bend those muscles and can't bend those knuckles.

As you think about closing your fingers to make a fist, your thoughts cause the fingers to grow progressively more stiff and rigid ... so stiff and rigid that you cannot make a fist. So think about moving your fingers and you find you cannot even bend your fingers. Stop trying.

As I gently rub your fingers, this causes your fingers to relax.

CLOSED FIST TEST

Extend your arms straight out from your chest and make a fist. Close those fingers tight ... tight ... still remaining deeply relaxed, I want you to open your eyes and look into my eyes.

I am going to count backward from five to one and each decreasing number causes your fingers to lock tighter and tighter ... so tight you won't be able to open your hand and stretch out your fingers.

Five ... fingers becoming clasped tight ... tight ... locked in place.

Four ... fingers locked tight.

Three ... fingers locking tighter, tighter and tighter.

Two ... fingers locking tight ... tight ...

And one ... fingers locked together so tight they will not separate and you cannot open your hand.

As you think about opening your fingers, your thoughts cause your fingers to grow stiff ... progressively more stiff and rigid ... so stiff and rigid that you cannot open your fingers. Stop trying.

Now as I touch your fingers, this causes your fingers to grow perfectly normal and you can open your fingers.

Arm Raising Test

I want you to concentrate now on your right arm as it gently rests on the arm of that chair.

As it remains there, your arm is starting to grow light ... light ... very light ... relaxing progressively more and more as it rests on the chair. It's growing so very light that it has no weight ... nothing to hold it down ... so very light.

It doesn't weigh as much as a feather ... the tiniest little feather and you have seen the tiniest little feather floating on the breeze, not enough weight to bring it down. The gentle breeze lifts it up ... up ... way up ...

Now your arm is light ... as light as that feather ... so very light ... so light, nothing can hold it down and feel it going up ... rising ... rising as a tiny feather rises up ... up it goes ... lifting ... lifting ...

Nothing can hold it down, nothing to keep it down ... rising up, up ... just as though there's a balloon up above and attached to the bottom of the balloon is a string and the string is attached to your wrist. As the balloon goes up ... up ... it lifts that tiny feather ... the wrist no heavier than a tiny feather ... up it goes ... rising ... rising up ... up ... nothing to hold it down ... up it goes ... it has no weight lifting higher and higher.

Now the balloon drifts over to your head ... up above your head as it moves over that way ... pulling the hand over toward your forehead and the hand moving closer and closer.

The moment it touches your forehead, it causes you to relax thoroughly and completely. Every muscle in your whole body lets go the moment your hand touches your forehead. The hand coming closer ... closer ... and closer and now it touches your forehead, causing every muscle in your whole body to let go and relax ... relaxing ... relaxing.

As I take your hand and gently lower your hand, it
restores the hand back to its normal weight. But the
lowering of the hand and arm causes your body to relax
even deeper and deeper ... going deeper and deeper as I
lower your hand, causing you to relax even deeper and
deeper ... deeply relaxing and letting go ... and relaxed.

HOT COIN TEST

For this test, the hypnotist needs a nickel or dime, a set of
tweezers, and a cigarette lighter. While the subject is seated with
the eyelids closed, hold the coin with the tweezers and then light
the lighter. Do not touch the lighter to the coin. Now speak to the
subject:

I want you to extend your arm straight out from
your shoulder, palm up. With your arm so extended and
still remaining deeply relaxed, I want you to open your
eyes and look at the coin. I am going to place the coin
on your hand and as the coin rests on your hand, you
feel it growing hotter and hotter ... and hotter ... so
hot that you cannot hold it.

(Release the coin from the tweezers onto the hand of the
subject.)

Now feel the coin growing hotter ... so hot it begins
to burn ... burning ... burning so hot that you cannot
hold it ... can't hold it at all. You have to drop it. Get rid
of it ... so very hot ... so very hot ... so very hot ... let
it go ... let it go.

CONFUSION TEST

I'm gently going to tap you on the forehead as I speak to you, so listen to each and every word that I have to say to you.

You ...

(Tap the subject on his forehead.)

... don't know your name. You ...

(Tap the subject on his forehead.)

... don't know your name. You ...

(Tap the subject on his forehead.)

... can't tell me your name. You ...

(Tap the subject on his forehead.)

... don't know who you are. Who are you? ... What's your name? ... You ...

(Tap the subject on his forehead.)

... don't know where you live. You ...

(Tap the subject on his forehead.)

... can't tell me where you live. Where do you live? ... What's your name? ... Where do you live? ... What's your name?

Amnesia of any other subject may be created in the same manner by gently tapping the subject on the forehead as you make a statement:

You don't know your name and don't know where you live. You don't know my name and don't know what day it is. You don't know where you are and don't know what city you live in.

Each and every time an adverse condition is created, it must be absolutely removed. The manner of removing amnesia is very simple. You may continue as follows:

I'm gently going to touch you on the forehead and gently rub your forehead and as I do so, each and every suggestion I gave you that "You don't know your name, don't know where you are" is now being erased. It is now erased. You have complete recall of everything and anything that you want to think about, no inhibitions any more. You are in complete control of everything.

(Then you may stop rubbing the subject's forehead).

ANESTHESIA

As you continue to sit in that chair, each passing moment causes you to relax even deeper and deeper and deeper.

And now it seems that your right leg is progressively relaxing more than the rest of your body. Your right leg from the hip all the way down to the toes is growing pleasantly more relaxed and more relaxed. Maybe even a numbness begins to set into that leg. Feel it growing pleasantly relaxed ... relaxed.

Accept that feeling of relaxation, comfort, and pleasure. All tension is leaving, dissipating, and flowing away as the leg progressively relaxes even more and more.

I'm going to gently touch you on the right knee with my finger and as I do, it causes that knee to become numb ...

(Touch the subject's knee with your finger.)

... growing progressively more numb ... useless ... and maybe even cold, and that numbness spreads deep into the knee, touching every muscle, every nerve, every fiber and cell, causing each of them to become numb and useless and maybe cold.

Now that numbness begins to spread from the knee down through each muscle and every nerve and cell ... all the way down to the ankle. As the numbness passes down through each nerve, it causes each nerve to become numb and useless and progressively more numb and useless down to the ankle.

That numbness now proceeds from the ankle into the foot and to your toes so that everything from the knee down to the toes is growing progressively more numb and useless as you continue to sit in this chair. Each passing moment causes that leg from the knee to the toes to grow progressively more numb ... absolutely useless ... and maybe even cold.

That numb feeling now begins to spread from the knee up through each muscle and every cell all the way to the hip, the whole leg growing numb and useless and maybe even cold ... absolutely numb and totally useless.

Yet you recognize you have a shoe on the end of the right foot. And the shoe seems to grow heavier and heavier, and the right leg grows more progressively numb. That shoe may feel like a boot, a heavy boot, like a heavy lead boot. The shoe may even feel like an anchor

... a heavy, heavy anchor ... like an anchor that is chained to the floor ... tightly chained to the floor. And that anchor is so very heavy and tightly chained to the floor, you cannot lift your right leg. For as you think about lifting the right leg, this causes the anchor to grow even heavier and heavier The leg is so totally useless, you can't lift the leg.

But go ahead and try to lift the leg and you find the anchor too heavy and the right leg so numb, you can't lift the leg. Try again but you can't.

I am going to take your right hand and place your hand on the thigh of that leg.

(Pick up the subject's hand and place it on the thigh of his right leg.)

All that numb feeling from the leg is now being absorbed into the right hand, and the right hand is growing progressively more numb and useless as the leg grows perfectly normal. All that feeling from the whole leg is being consolidated into that small hand, causing it to become absolutely numb, totally useless, and maybe cold. Each passing moment causes the hand to become progressively more useless ... absolutely numb and maybe totally useless and maybe cold ... cold and useless. As you continue to concentrate on that right hand, it causes that hand to become progressively more useless, progressively more numb ... maybe cold, your leg growing perfectly normal in every respect while the right hand becomes absolutely numb, totally useless.

Now I'm going to pick up that right hand very
gently by the wrist and lift the whole arm up ... nice and
easy ... and now I'm placing the right hand on the left
shoulder, causing the shoulder to become totally numb
and completely useless. All that feeling is now moving
from the hand into the left shoulder, and the shoulder is
growing absolutely numb and totally useless as the hand
grows perfectly normal. As that feeling is transferred, it
increases in its intensity of numbness and uselessness ...
the shoulder becoming totally numb and completely
useless. As you concentrate on the left shoulder ...
every nerve growing absolutely numb and totally useless
... no feeling whatsoever ... none whatsoever.

The created feeling of anesthesia may be transferred from
the leg to the hand and then from the hand to any portion or part of
the body by merely taking the hand and placing it in position. Should
you be unable to reach and touch any part of the body, such as the
lower back or some part that is inaccessible, then all you have to
do is continue as follows:

Now your hand is totally and completely and
absolutely numb and totally useless. I'm going to reach
down to the wrist of your hand, and I will grasp that
feeling just as though I am grasping a rag. The feeling is
a rag in your hand ... a rag of numbness and
uselessness. I am gently going to bring my hand up from
your wrist up to your elbow, dragging that feeling
through each muscle ... bringing that feeling of
numbness and uselessness all the way up to the elbow.

Now you can feel it as it comes through the elbow up to the shoulder ... dragging that feeling of numbness and uselessness right through your arm, right to your shoulder, and across your shoulder and down your back. Now down into the lower back that feeling of numbness and uselessness now touches every muscle, every nerve, and every cell in your lower back ... spreading deep ... deep into that area, causing everything to become numb ... and totally and absolutely useless ... no feeling in that back ... absolutely numb and totally useless ... and it will stay that way until I remove it.

You cannot take it away ... only I can remove it. You cannot take it away ... only I can remove it. I put it there and I will be the only one that can take it away ... remaining there always in a numb and useless manner until I remove it.

So accept the feeling of comfort and relaxation as it settles deep, deep in the back, bringing you comfort, satisfaction, and relief ... relief from tension, apprehension, and discomfort. So let it stay ... soothing and further relaxing the whole area, making you feel more comfortable, more pleasant, more relaxed ... and life more enjoyable. Accept that feeling of relaxation and numbness deep in the muscles.

In the event there is a pain in the lower back that should be removed, then you can describe that feeling in the hand as being a white blanket or something very comforting like a piece of wool, but make sure it's white, pleasant, and wonderful. Then describe the area of the pain as being colored with a dark piece of cloth or a small black blanket. Take the white blanket and put it into the area where the dark blanket is. Then grasp the dark blanket and proceed to follow the same course from the back up to the shoulder, down the arm, and put the dark and dirty feeling of pain into the hand. What you're doing, in effect, is exchanging the numbness from the hand to the back, and the discomfort and pain from the back to the hand. Now all of the pain is in the hand. Then continue in this manner:

> On the end of your fingers of your hand, there are tiny valves and I'm asking those valves to slowly open. And as I rub your hand, it causes the dark material to change into dark liquid and the liquid then gently drips … drips through the ends of your fingers, taking with it all that dark feeling of discomfort and tension.

> Just let that discomfort seep through your fingertips and when all of that feeling is gone, the valves will automatically close by themselves. And your hand becomes perfectly comfortable and pleasantly relaxed. I want you to let me know when all of that dark feeling is gone and the valves are closed by gently nodding your head YES, IT'S ALL GONE.

(The subject's head nods.)

> That's fine. Now, I just want you to relax … pleasantly relaxing. Let yourself go deeper into relaxation with each passing moment … so just relax and enjoy that feeling of pleasure and comfort and satisfaction.

POSITIVE HALLUCINATIONS

While you have been sitting here during this session, my little cat came into this room and is right next to the chair you are occupying. I know from our previous discussion during the interview that you like cats. So still remaining deeply relaxed, open your eyes and look down at the cat.

(The subject opens his eyes and looks down.)

Why don't you reach down and pet the cat and then pick it up and put it in your lap?

(The subject pets and picks up the cat.)

Since my neighbor gave me this cat, I am not sure just how old the cat is. So why don't you examine it and tell me how old you think it is?

(The subject responds.)

Put the cat down on the floor and close your eyes and just let yourself relax ... going deeper and deeper into relaxation.

Or another dialogue may be this:

Just a few minutes ago a person came into this room and this person said that you are friends; however, I am not quite sure that is the case. Although this person is a friend of mine, I'm not really sure you know this person.

In a moment, I am going to have you open your eyes so you can tell me whether or not you know this person. And if you do, tell me this person's name and how you came to know this person. If you don't know this

person, just say that you don't and I will clap my hands
like this ...

(Clap your hands.)

... and a cloud of smoke will surround this person.
And then both the person and the cloud of smoke will
just disappear.

Now, still remaining deeply relaxed, open your eyes
and look over to the couch and describe this person.

At the time the eyes are opened, the hypnotist should watch
for any particular facial expressions for clues leading to hallucinatory expressions.

Although no cat entered the room, the subject in somnambulism does "see" this cat when the suggestions are made in a
positive manner, leading the subject to believe there is a cat in the
room. Instead of a cat, the hypnotist may suggest that a book, lamp,
picture, or any other object has just been brought into the room for
the subject to describe. These expressions by the subject will permit
the hypnotist to determine whether or not the subject's reactions
are real or whether he is just going along with the hypnotist's
suggestions to please the hypnotist.

In those cases where hallucinatory suggestions are applied
to a person, do not attempt to describe the person or make any
reference to the sex of the person. Should the subject recognize the
person, inquire further as to the manner of dress, how they became
acquainted, where the person lives, or any other facts about the
person. Then the subject is asked to close his eyes and the imaginary
person is asked to leave the room.

When the person is not recognized by the subject, then the
hypnotist claps his hands, creating the smoke and causing the person
to disappear. Usually a confused and frightened expression will
appear on the face of the subject when the person disappears in the
cloud of smoke, so it is necessary to assure the subject that the
person never really existed but the image was only an illusion.

Negative Hallucinations

While the subject is in a state of hypnosis, place three or four objects (such as a book, glass, ashtray, or pencil) on a nearby table. When these objects are placed, then describe only three of them to the subject with the statement that there are only three objects on the table. Then continue as follows:

I have placed three objects on the table here in this room. These three are a book, an ashtray, and a pencil. These things are on this table, and I have removed all other objects so that these three are the only things on this table.

Now, still remaining pleasantly relaxed, open your eyes and look over there at the table and describe these three objects to me. As you look at these objects, please tell me which one is on the right side and which one is on the left side and which one is in the middle.

Since I haven't placed anything else on the table, I want you to go over to the table and pick up everything you see and bring them over to me.

The statement that these three objects are the only things on the table and all other objects have been removed is the key to the condition of negative hallucination. When the subject is in a deep state of hypnosis, the only things that will be seen are those described.

Inability to Speak

I have found creating a condition where the subject is unable to speak, to be one of the most effective tests and a method of convincing the subject that hypnosis has been created. When a person is satisfied that he has been hypnotized, then every therapeutic suggestion is accepted with open arms and enthusiasm. When this test has been conducted successfully, behavioral changes follow almost as a matter of course. Successful treatment is within reach.

However, this test requires patience, skill, and timing. Once the language commences, it should be delivered in a smooth, continuous voice, unhurried and uninterrupted. The continuous delivery does not allow time for the subject to analyze the impact of the statements being made. The statements incorporated in the suggestions are then passively accepted and for this individual, they are true. Once these suggestions, true or false, are recorded within the memory bank, the subject's response is then predictable.

The test starts exactly the same as that outlined in creating anesthesia of the leg. Once the feeling of numbness and uselessness is created and the subject is unable to lift the leg, then the hand is placed on the thigh, absorbing that feeling like a sponge. Don't assume that the hand automatically absorbs this feeling but create the condition by suggestion.

Now I am going to pick up that arm and lift up that useless and numb hand.

(Place one hand between the elbow and shoulder, and the other at the wrist; then lift the arm, allowing the hand to hang limply.)

Now I am going to lift up that numb and useless hand and place the hand on your neck, causing this numb and useless feeling to flow gently down into your neck.

(Still holding the arm, let the hand gently touch the neck.)

This numbness is now being absorbed by the neck muscles, causing them to be numb and useless.

(Gently rub the neck with the hand.)

As I gently rub your neck with the hand, this causes the numbness to flow and spread into the jaw muscles, the chin, and into the lips. This feeling of numbness now flows down between the lips into your mouth and down your throat, touching the vocal cords, causing them to become numb and useless, so numb and useless that you cannot speak one word, not one word.

I am going to ask you some questions and you know all the answers. As you think about the answers to my questions, your thoughts cause cotton balls to form in your throat, causing your lips to grow numb and useless and your lips to turn to wax, thick heavy wax.

But go ahead and think about the answers to my questions, and you find that you cannot say one word. Not one word. Why, you cannot even tell me your first name. But go ahead and think about your first name, but you cannot speak ...
(Wait for a few seconds, then continue.)

You can't tell me what city you live in. I know you know what city you live in, but you can't tell me the city ...
(Wait a few more seconds.)

You can't tell me the kind of vehicle you drove here and I know you know what vehicle you drove to come here. But go ahead and think of the name of the vehicles and try to tell me the name of the vehicle.

Why, you can't even tell me the name of the person who came with you today. But think of the person's

name and try to tell the name you find, but you cannot
even talk.

Watch the subject very closely. When there is some
noticeable movement of the lips or a straining of the neck muscles
in an attempt to speak, then the subject may be challenged. Do not
challenge the subject unless there is an assurance of success.

I am now going to gently place my hand on your
forehead and as I do so ...

(Place your hand on the subject's forehead.)

... it causes your neck muscles to become perfectly
normal, your lips normal, and your vocal cords perfectly
normal so you can now speak with ease and comfort.
You speak better now than before, for your diction is
excellent and your enunciation perfect. Why, the words
just flow out so simply and so easy. So go ahead and tell
me your name.

(Remove your hand from the subject's forehead.)

10

DEVELOPING THE IMMUNE SYSTEM

Pain, suffering, and depression become secondary when the patient or subject is suffering from a severe, debilitating, or terminal disease. In most patients, a time pattern of psychic death has been established and formulated so that death may be predicted within months of the origin of the diagnosis. The attending physician is always on guard for the inevitable question: "How long do I have to live?" When the answer is not straightforward, the patient will interpret the evasive answer into meaning that his remaining days are rather short. At this point, the patient is overcome with fear, loneliness, depression, and self-pity together with an underlying delayed reaction of hatred.

Since there are no known cures for cancer and other terminal diseases, treatment is delayed for fear that the condition is already beyond repair. Early detection and removal or treatment can and will reward the patient with additional years of productive and enjoyable life. However, when the words indicating terminal diseases are spoken, there is an immediate deterioration of the thought process, resulting in negative body responses.

At the mere mention of cancer and having accepted the fact that he is suffering from such a disease, the patient begins the downward progress, resulting in death within the limits of the time prescribed or mentioned by the attending physician. The conscious mind now works in unison with the subconscious mind to create the inevitable result of early death. The thought *I cannot survive* becomes deeply embedded in the memory bank, preventing its removal by conscious effort. The conscious mind has the ability to feed the information into the memory bank but lacks the capacity to remove any thought that has been placed there and becomes deeply embedded within. The removal of the thoughts is limited to the powers of the subconscious mind. Returning back to the basic principle that it is the subconscious mind that directs the brain to perform in any manner, we can now begin to recognize how corrective suggestions may be implemented.

Consider for a moment a patient who has just been informed that he is suffering from colon cancer of some duration. His immediate backlash thought is: *I am condemned to an early death.* Every ache and pain thereafter are accepted by the patient to mean the condition is worsening, and any assurances by his physician that these pains are not related are rejected. With the passing days and months, the patient retreats within himself and develops symptoms of self-pity, depression, hatred, and loneliness, causing him to become entirely dependent upon family and other relatives for the ordinary daily chores. When this dependency becomes overbearing upon the family, especially with no hopeful future in sight, the repressed desire for an early demise begins to settle within the individuals most concerned.

Overcoming the torment that by now has undermined the patient is a very difficult and almost impossible for the hypnotist. The patient must first be convinced there is room for hope, and a commitment must be made to survive against insurmountable odds. The dreaded feeling of death is ever-present. The helpless and lost sensation within must be overcome, and the question, "How can I succeed and cure myself when all of the best medicine provides no hope?" must be answered in a convincing manner. Years of scientific research have failed to provide an encouraging answer; however, research in clinical hypnosis and the small measure of success give hope where no hope previously existed.

Every doctor has heard mysterious stories of a patient's recovery from a disease that denied conventional explanation. Such stories give rise to the doctrine that there exists some undefined element to healing that is not subject to microscopic examination or laboratory tests. Some element in the mind of the patient makes a very important contribution in regard to the difference of that person's reactions to illness. Whatever happens in the mind also happens in the body.

During the early stages of development of modern medicine, immunologists concluded the immune system was autonomous in nature, functioning independently from the rest of the body's organs. However, around 1950 researchers learned the immune system could tell which cells belonged to the body and which were foreign cells, that the immune system possessed a biochemical memory that helped it recognize and destroy certain cells, and that it was capable of sending millions of killer cells to assist in this destruction. One encounter of a foreign cell was sufficient for future recognition.

Continued research and laboratory studies revealed other very interesting and disturbing patterns of conduct. Not only is the immune system called upon to locate, identify, and destroy cells entering the body through external avenues, but it is also required to destroy and remove cells affected by functional stress arising during everyday activities.

Ductless glands, for example, such as the adrenal and pituitary glands, release their powerful secretions directly into the bloodstream in such varying amounts as may be necessary. Since the brain runs, rules, and controls the function of each cell in the body, we must therefore recognize that it is the brain that causes the condition to start or stop.

In each and every stressful or traumatic situation, the body undergoes a number of changes. Some situations will produce a combination of changes such as increased pulse rate, sweating, nervousness, shortness of breath, or any other emotional response such as fight or flight. It is therefore concluded that if stress or a traumatic event can create such an immediate response, then shouldn't some other factor within be able to turn it off? These are only some of the clues linking the brain to the immune system. The next question, then, begs for an answer. If the brain can influence the immune system, is there some way we can control and direct this function of the brain? The answer to this is yes.

Assume for a moment that two individuals were just concluding a conversation in a closed room and one of them was leaving. As he opened the door to leave, he was confronted with a tall, heavy individual wearing dirty clothes and a gun pointed directly at him. The normal reaction would be for him to feel an increase in pulse rate, accelerated breathing, sweating, and anticipation of physical harm. The fight-or-flight syndrome would begin to manifest itself. Without any words spoken, the body changes were immediately caused by what he saw. Accompanying this image was the perception it gave, and the mind analyzing these factors concluded this was a dangerous and stressful situation.

The events unfolded so quickly, the person was not consciously aware of his physical changes. However, upon hearing the remark, "Don't worry, he is only a friend of mine returning my gun," the body instantly undergoes further changes, reflecting the concept that this dangerous condition never really existed. Although the physical facts remain the same (that of the man holding the gun), the person's thoughts of the situation changed, resulting in emotional and physical changes. The only difference in the entire picture is the thinking.

We previously recognized that there was a relationship between the brain and the immune system, and now we can add the third element: the psycho – how we think. Putting the three together, we have the *psycho* (state of mind), *neuro* (brain), and *immunology* (the immune system). Hence, the word "psycho-neuroimmunology."

Brain cells are called neurons and are located within and protected by the skull, communicating with one another by means of neurotransmitters. Each neuron is capable of transmitting and receiving thousands of messages at any given moment. These messages fall within one of two categories:

1. Excitatory, to do something
2. Inhibitory, to stop doing something

During normal circumstances, these messages are equal in number, allowing the person to enjoy a calm and controlled attitude; however, when the messages are out of balance, the result may be overactive or depressive. After these messages are transferred from brain cell to brain cell, they travel along fine, hair-like fibers called nerves to their ultimate destination in the particular organ or cell.

The immune system is a complicated, organized group of cells that have their own system of communication and alert each cell of the condition of other cells in the body. They have their origin in the bone marrow and follow different pathways of development. About one half of these cells are carried by the bloodstream to the thymus gland, the source of powerful hormones that allow the newly created cells to mature into powerful T-cells.

There are several types of T-cells. The helper T-cell is the most important T-cell. The helper T-cell has a memory bank of one million antigens, things that can destroy or harm the body. Upon recognizing any antigen, the helper T-cell instantly secretes a biochemical substance that alerts other immune system cells into action to locate, identify, destroy, and remove the antigen from the body.

Other cells that make up a part of the immune system are the B-cells, natural killer cells, killer T-cells, suppressor T-cells, lymphocytes, phagocytes, macrophages, and null cells (just to name a few). These by no means comprise the entire system. These cells functioning alone would be entirely ineffective in combating disease or destroying tumor tissue.

Some of the glands in the immune system are the thymus, bone marrow, lymph nodes, and hypothalamus (just to name a few of these). The hypothalamus is a giant drug factory, producing stress-sensitive hormones that, in turn, cause norepinephrine, epinephrine, and corticosteroids to be produced, each of which has a definite effect on the immune system.

Now we come to where the hypnotist plays an important part in the chain of events within. The most important ingredient in psychoneuroimmunology (PNI) is the psycho, the mind. All other segments are organic and like all organic matters in the whole body, they respond to commands, instructions, and orders. Some of these are preprogrammed by our very nature and the inherent natural law of survival, while others emerge from our activities and environments.

In this whole scheme of existence, we tend to lose sight of the two major premises:

1. Nothing is accomplished unless or until it is preceded by a thought, either current or previously established.
2. The brain rules and controls each and every cell in the body.

Research has taught us that the brain's connecting nerve tissues run through every gland (such as the thymus, lymph nodes, and spleen) that makes up a large part of the function of the immune system. No major or minor sector of the immune system is without a direct connection to the brain.

Various states of mind and our acceptance or rejection of the feeling or symptom, resulting from the creation of the state of mind, can result in a biochemical aftershock consistent with the severity of the state of mind. We act or we react not always to the true nature of an event but to how we perceive it to be. If time would permit us to analyze or reason as the events unfold, our state of mind – that is, how we accept or reject circumstances – would differ and our actions might take a different course.

Stress, for example, is a state of mind and most of the brain's effect on the health of any individual comes from the degree of stress sustained. During any stressful situation, a tiny pituitary gland affixed at the base of the brain releases endorphines, a powerful brain drug, into the bloodstream. Any kind of stress, regardless of the nature of its origin, instantly creates a release of the painkillers into the blood. These painkillers attempt to neutralize the stressful situation so that one is able to cope with the present circumstances. As circumstances change, so will the state of mind.

Unfortunately, the longer an individual allows the stressful situation to exist, the more troublesome it becomes. And the longer our attempts to cope with the situation end up in failure, the more desperate becomes the state of mind. Eventually it will give up all further attempts and accept failure, rendering the situation permanent and creating an emotional fallout of worry and fear. The hypnotist can, and must, create a state of mind that can successfully cope with the stressful situation.

When worry and fear are allowed to remain, it may lead to loss of appetite and social inactivity and eventually total helplessness. By now, we must realize that a person is continuously bombarded with two methods of attack – emotional and physical. Whichever comes first, the other is soon to follow. Should an individual suffer cancerous tumors, he usually becomes so emotionally stressed-out, his body surrenders itself to all other diseases. On the other hand, when a person is faced with a stressful situation and he accepts the attitude that he can't cope with it, he allows the helpless and hopeless state of mind to take charge, surrendering all effort to cope, thereby succumbing to illness and physical problems. Stress is a component in every disease, and the removal of stress by the hypnotist lessens one very important ingredient in the physical ailment.

The immune system basically has two means for defending the body:

1. One is the humoral immunity, which depends on special molecules always present in the bloodstream. These antibodies are able to move quickly to the site of the infection or injury.
2. The other is cell-mediated immunity, which utilizes a team of cells to inform the immune system of the presence of virus or bacteria and then organizes an attack on it.

It is to the cell-mediated immunity that the hypnotist must direct his suggestions. These cells work in conjunction with responses to activity of other cells. They are instructed to respond, based upon the conduct of other cells in direct line of communication.

Consider for a moment the activity of this cell-mediated immunity. Constantly on patrol are the cells that make up the immune system. Each one of us has approximately four billion such cells. However, each day we lose a billion and each day we grow another billion. When an immune cell encounters a foreign bacterium, it splits off a molecule and carries this molecule to the helper T-cell for identification. The helper T-cell has a memory bank of one million antigens, things that can destroy or harm the body. Upon identification that the bacterium is harmful, the helper T-cell discharges a biochemical substance into the body, alerting the system of the presence of this bacterium.

The B-cells, ever present near the lymph glands, pick up this warning and, in turn, release into the blood stream antibodies particular to that bacteria. Once these antibodies reach the bacteria, they attack, invade, and attempt to isolate it by forming a coating over it. When the antibody discharged by the B-cell is in the body, this alerts the reserve or backup cells. The natural killer cells, killer T-cells, phagocytes, the null cells, and the other cells comprising the reserve system go into action. The reserve cells, in turn, attack the bacteria and engage in a battle to destroy the bacteria.

When the bacteria have been destroyed, then the suppressor T-cells send out their own biochemical substance calling off the attack and requesting the cells to return to their specific glands until the next encounter. In the meantime, the phagocytes and the macrophages clean up the residue and cart the residue to the urine and stool. One encounter with that particular bacteria, or enemy, and the cells retain a memory of their potential destruction. Should another encounter take place, instantly a battle erupts.

Each step in the function of the immune system is a well-organized and intelligent process with a specific goal to be accomplished. Every such attack follows a precisely described routine. To organize takes planning, and planning takes intelligence. So where does this intelligence originate?

The only source of this thought process is the mind – that elusive, intangible energy. At the moment of conception, this vast knowledge directing the immune system is passed from one generation to the next. However, during the lifetime of an individual, there is a constant bombardment of interrupting and disturbing thoughts that can affect the function of this system. When the incoming thoughts, impressions or impulses become overwhelming, the immune system breaks down and the person is unable to destroy the virus or bacteria within. Drugs must then be injected into the body to aid in destroying the enemy. The longer the immune system is permitted to continue its inefficient course, the more permanent it becomes, and this inefficiency is passed along to the next generation. This new generation then "inherits" the disease of past generations needlessly.

Control of each cell and the function thereof rest with the brain. However, the brain refuses to act until it has been directed and has received a command to perform. The decision to perform may be on the conscious level, but performance is on the subconscious level. This control center is intricately connected by a vast network of nerves relaying messages for action or inaction. The origin of any message must be the result of a thought process. To conclude otherwise would be to assume that the brain creates the thoughts and directs their performance. Following this line of reasoning, it would then be fair to conclude that each of us would, under similar circumstances, perform identically as our brains function in a precise pattern.

The only thing that makes each of us different is how we think. A group of ten individuals faced with an unexpected event will respond in ten different ways, each following his own thoughts and perceptions. We are genetically and immunologically different: genetically different due to the acceptance or rejection of thoughts, impressions, and impulses on our parents and their predecessors; immunologically different due to the influences of diet, sex, race, state of mind, attitude, and our ability to deal with a stressful situation (just to name a few factors).

We must accept the PNI theory that there is a connection between the mind and the immune system, otherwise the thought process is irrelevant to that of the rest of the body. We already know certain states of mind – that is, how we perceive a situation to be – do have a powerful biochemical influence. The more we research, the more we realize our body does respond to how we think.

States of mind have a decided effect on glands and their chemical-producing ability. A stressful state of mind affects the hypothalamus and its ability to produce hormones which are vital to the immune system. Other states of mind cause other reactions, varying in degree of effect on the immune system. The longer a negative, depressive state continues to exist, the more influence it has on the immune system. Giving up, for example, is a complete surrender of the immune system to disease. The loss of hope, realistic or otherwise, means death is near.

Since the brain is connected to every cell, diseased or otherwise, any message to the brain from the subconscious mind is immediately relayed to each cell. Instructions by the hypnotist must be directed to both the diseased cell and the cells of the immune system. I must repeat, for emphasis, that the brain controls each cell and it receives its commands, orders, and instructions from the subconscious mind which, in turn, is relayed to the cell, causing the cells to respond accordingly.

Credibility is the most important word in utilizing the immune system to treat the patient in the state of hypnosis. Nothing can be accomplished unless the patient believes in the treatment, so the hypnotist's first obligation is to educate the patient in what he is trying to accomplish and how he will go about doing it. This requires the hypnotist to have a certain amount of knowledge of the function of the immune system and the ability to explain this function in such terms that the average patient will understand it. Treatment begins with the interview and the rapport that is developed during the session. As trust in the hypnotist grows, so does the patient's responsiveness.

Conduct a general conversation with the subject relative to the information provided by the subject on the data sheet, prepared by the subject before the first session. Direct the conversation into the area of hypnosis by seeking out the subject's knowledge and impressions of hypnosis, and then give your explanation of hypnosis and why it works for the subject's benefit. When the hypnotist is satisfied that the subject has a good grasp of hypnosis, the method by which the immune system functions should be explained without going into a lengthy, detailed discussion. Unless the subject is acquainted with the immune system, it may be difficult to create some imagery of the cells engaged in battle. The use of a chalkboard with some sketching of the cells is usually helpful. When drawing the various cells, always make the immune cells larger than the diseased cells; for this pre-instructs the subject to imagine such cells as being stronger and more powerful.

The subject is now ready to be hypnotized by any method of induction that the hypnotist may elect with the progressive relaxation and two deepening techniques following. I prefer to use the "counting backward from one to one hundred" method, followed by the alphabet technique (as outlined in Chapter 11). Testing for depth may be attempted at this time only if the outward appearance of the subject shows he is thoroughly relaxed. No attempt to test the subject should ever be made unless the hypnotist expects a positive response. In the event that the test provides a negative response, all further tests should be terminated and alternative deepening techniques administered, allowing the subject to further relax, physically and mentally. Under these circumstances, recognize that the subject is either too resistant or exceptionally apprehensive, so the session should be ended. Arrange for a subsequent session at which time the proper depth may be achieved.

When the subject is ready to the satisfaction of the hypnotist for suggestive therapy, the subject should be taken down to the library. He is then age-regressed by taking him down the aisle between the bookshelves to a time preceding the present ailment. Following the procedure previously outlined, the books representing the present difficulties are removed from the shelves, thrown away, and removed from the library, the memory bank. These books may have such titles as *Cancer, Pain, Lung Disease, Headaches, I Can't, Excuses*, or any other that may be indicative of the subject's problems. Once the books have been removed and the subject is seated in the comfortable library chair experiencing a feeling of complete relaxation, he is ready for the suggestions as may be necessary for the improvement of his immune system.

Continue as follows:

You recall earlier we talked about the immune system and how the various cells communicated with one another to destroy damaged cells. These immune system cells are permanently patrolling your body looking for viruses, germs, bacteria, and troubled areas in your body. Remember that when these patrolling cells encounter an invader, a cell that doesn't belong in your body, or discover a cell that you built that turned out to be confused, mutated, or diseased, these cells must then, in turn, be destroyed. Some of the diseased cells cover themselves with a coating material to disguise themselves to look like good cells. Sometimes your immune system cells get lazy and don't patrol as efficiently as they should. So now it's time for you to instruct these patrolling cells to be more efficient.

Walk around in this library of yours and as you walk around, you do find a door that is open. When you see the open door, just nod your head YES so I know that you have found the open door.

(The patient nods his head.)

Now look around some more and not too far from the open door, there is a door that is closed. Again, when you see the closed door, nod your head YES so I know you have found the closed door.

(The patient nods his head.)

Let me tell you what is behind the closed door.

When you were born and still a tiny wet baby, the Almighty stood over you and spread His hands over your body and blessed you. These blessings landed on your body and covered your whole body like angel dust, starlets, or sprinkles. These blessings entered into your body through the tiny pores in your skin and became living cells.

These cells patrol your entire body looking for, finding, and destroying viruses, bacteria, germs, and foreign material that enter into your body. The doctors call these cells your immune and defensive system. I prefer to call these cells workers, protectors, friends, helpers, even soldiers and angels. For most of your life, these friends, helpers, and protectors were very efficient and kept your body free from disease and discomfort. But somewhere and somehow you insulted your friends, workers, and protectors.

You see, each and every time you criticized yourself, you also criticized your workers and helpers. And so too every time you became stressed, you also stressed your friends, workers, and helpers and they became lazy. The more you became stressed and the more you have criticized yourself, the lazier and more inefficient they became.

You have reached a point that your workers, helpers, friends, and protectors got so disgusted, they threw up their hands and said, "If you don't care, why should we work so hard?"

When they became so disgusted, they went behind the closed door and remained there.

Understand that your problem developed because your friends, workers, and helpers were no longer protecting your body. So with your permission, I am going to get the door open and instruct your workers, helpers, protectors, friends, maybe soldiers and angels to go back to work and do the job that the Almighty intended for them to do.

Do you want the door opened? If you do, just nod your head YES so I know that you want the door open. (The patient nods his head.)

Always ask for permission to have the door opened. When permission is given, that is reassurance that the person is motivated to recovery. In all the years that I have been in hypnosis, only once did the subject not express the desire to have the door opened. Later, I found out that she had suicidal tendencies. In this case, I told her it was my moral duty to have the door opened and I told her that when I clap my hands together, this causes the door to burst wide open. I clapped my hands very hard without any hesitation. Much to her surprise, the door just fell apart. I then instructed her that the door was so broken that no one could put it together. Not only was the door broken but also her depression. She fully recovered.

Continue as follows:

I am gently going to place my hand on your forehead and the moment I touch your forehead, this causes the closed door to burst wide open and when the door is open, out come your workers, helpers, and protectors in a never ending number, like an army into the library and then out the open door and back into your body to do the work they were initially intended to do.

Now keep your eyes on the closed door.

(Gently place your hand on the forehead with the thumb on one temple and a finger on the other temple.)

Now the door has burst open and it's shattered and out come your protectors, helpers, friends, and maybe soldiers and angels in a never ending number into the library and then out the opened door and back into your body. I can't see them but you can. Don't be surprised how they look.

When you see your workers, helpers, protectors, just nod your head YES.

(The patient nods his head.)

In the next chapter on hypnotherapy, I state that when the subject sees the bookshelves in rows, the subject will see everything after that. So when you state that the workers and protectors come out the door, expect the subject to see this happen. Why it works is not important, just know it works. I explained beforehand that when I place my hand on the forehead, the door will burst wide open and the workers come out. If you want a person to see something specific, you must explain ahead of time what is going to happen and then the subject realizes those expectations.

Continue as follows:

Now your workers, helpers, protectors, friends, soldiers and maybe angels work for you. Your thoughts are their commands and instructions. These thoughts that you give are relayed by the brain through all of the wires called nerves to the workers and helpers, causing them to perform the duties that you request.

I am going to ask your friends and workers to patrol your entire body from the top of the head, all the way down to your toes and to the ends of your fingertips and examine each and every cell in your whole body. To look for, search, examine each cell, tissue, gland, and organ for any foreign material such as viruses, bacteria, germs, and chemicals that are harmful and dangerous to your body. To identify these invaders and destroy the viruses, germs, bacteria, and chemicals and remove the residue to the stool and urine so you can expel this out of your body.

I am also going to ask your friends, workers, and protectors to search for, locate, and identify any diseased tissue, tumors, cluster of cells and any cells that are present in the body that do not perform any useful healthy function in the body. To destroy these unnecessary and harmful cells and tissues. To look for cells that should be soft and when these cells have a hard exterior, to destroy the cells and remove the interior material down to the stool and urine.

This is when the workers and helpers are directed to a specific area in the body where the doctors have indicated there is a tumor or tumors, infected tissues, or suspected problems. You may also ask the patient to touch certain areas specifically locating the tumors or infected tissues. The therapist should never touch unless he has permission and the area is not personal. The more specific the instructions and the more detailed the area is described, the more success you can expect.

Continue as follows:

I am also asking the brain to collapse the veins and capillaries that serve the tumors, infected tissues, and cancer cells and stop serving these tissues with the energy to keep the tissues, cancer cells, and tumors alive. To allow these cells to die immediately.

It is necessary to kill these cells that are harmful and dangerous for survival of the body. I am also asking the brain to continue this process of searching, locating, and destroying these tumors, cancer cells and tissues until the process is complete, destroying all of the tumors, cancer cells and tissue that serve no useful function, until the body is fully healed and healthy.

Nothing is beyond the power of your subconscious mind to aid in the recovery of your body. The imprints, instructions, and suggestions that you have given are now permanently recorded in your Health and Happiness, Success, and Desire books and continue to direct your helpers, workers, protectors, friends, soldiers, and maybe angels in keeping your body protected from cancer cells and invaders.

Be proud of who you are. Give yourself credit for taking the time to heal yourself. Look after your precious body. It's the only one you are going to have, so love yourself. Be pleased with yourself and do not let anyone harm you or cause any physical or mental injury. Protect yourself even from your own harmful acts.

Now is the time to leave your library, your sanctuary, your retreat, and return to the conscious state of awareness. I am going to count from one to three, and at the count of three, your eyelids do open and you are alert and feeling wonderful, relaxed, comfortable, and satisfied in mind and body.

One ... two ... and three.

The foregoing language should be delivered very slowly and methodically. Take your time. Pause between each sentence. Let the subject or patient absorb each descriptive word. Allow time for the patient to grasp the meaning of such words and permit him sufficient time to formulate a picture or image in his mind of each thing you are describing.

A sentence should be delivered in this manner:

Close by ... or nearby ... there is another door and it's closed ... find this door ... you can see it ... when you see this door ... again ... nod your head YES ...

Whenever a patient is able to visualize the bookshelves in the library, he will be able to find the doors and his protectors. Do not attempt to describe the protectors, workers, helpers, or friends. Each patient's description will vary, so do not attempt to put one patient's description into another patient's image or picture. It just doesn't work.

Due to the varying types of the immune system, I prefer to use several terms, such as *soldiers, workers, helpers, friends, protectors*, and maybe *angels*. Each of these descriptive words carries a separate and distinct connotation in the minds of the subjects. *Soldiers* may mean people who would not hesitate to protect or carry out a command; they are duty bound. *Workers* are those who go about and methodically get the job done. *Helpers* are those who assist because there is a need for assistance. *Friends* are those who get the work done because they are ready to help. *Protectors* are guardians and *angels* enhance one's belief in the Almighty, whose power is universal and unlimited.

Keep interchanging the words by referring to the immune system as being soldiers and helpers, and then another time as being workers and friends. By interchanging these words, we begin to mold all of the characteristics into one figure, ending up with an individual object that is strong, very friendly, and a good worker.

Following the session, ask the patient to describe the immune system or workers. Make a note on his chart as to just how the patient views his system for future reference. Show no surprise and do not make fun of the description the patient gives. Over the years, I have heard the immune system called Pac-man, Dow Chemical Cleaners, Scrubbies, Brushes, Arrows, Shovels, Fish, Cotton Balls, Large and Small Soldiers, Those on Horses, and Little People (to name a few). The clothing, uniforms, and dress vary in color.

Recently one of my cancer patients described them as being Grains of Rice. At the subsequent session, he explained the rice concept. In his mind, they were kernels and he was a retired colonel in the Air Force. The words *kernel* and *colonel* are pronounced the same. At the time that he first created the image of his immune system, he was not aware of the close association of the two words. It was during a self-hypnosis session that he recognized the similarity. This brought a pleased smile to his face as this recognition led to a feeling of security, of being in the hands of superior officers.

It is the brain that causes the body to function. The thought is the energy and impulse to the brain requesting certain action, and upon receipt of this instruction, the brain then commences the process of body action. The brain, on its own, cannot cause any action. The initial and motivating force must come from the thought process.

In a state of hypnosis – that is, in a state of awareness dominated by the subconscious mind – body functions may be altered, changed, and modified by suggestion. Upon acceptance of the suggestion by the subject or patient, the brain either causes some action to happen or prevents the function of what we would consider ordinary and normal. Most of us consider the ability to speak a normal and ordinary body function; however, by proper suggestion, speaking can be entirely removed or modified. Since we speak with no conscious effort, we must then assume this body function is controlled by the subconscious mind. So if the subconscious mind can cause a change, then we must recognize that the subconscious mind can direct the brain to increase or decrease all functions in the body. Through the use of hypnosis, bodily functions such as breathing, walking, running, sitting down, standing up, hearing, smelling, or any number of other functions can be altered or entirely inhibited.

During one of my party demonstrations, I asked a young lady in a state of hypnosis if she would like a drink of water, since she was thirsty. At her request, she was given a glass of cool liquid and when she had finished drinking, I said to her in a surprised voice that I made a mistake and had given her a glass of gin. Immediately, she started to cough and became extremely upset, thinking she had consumed a full glass of gin. This was followed by a suggestion that she would become intoxicated and would need some assistance in getting home. Within a few minutes, she began exhibiting signs of intoxication and in less than an hour, she passed out on a couch. Once she had not rejected the suggestion that what she had consumed was gin, the responsive conduct was an automatic process over which she had no control.

Such is the effect of the subconscious mind upon the body functions. It is not material to the subconscious mind whether or not the statements and suggestions are true. It is the intended effect, by the language used, that causes the subconscious mind to respond the way it does.

11

HYPNOTHERAPY

The procedures and techniques outlined in this chapter are what I use several times a day. The more often these techniques are practiced, the more successful you become. Each and every subject (patient) goes through exactly the same procedures until the suggestive therapy is utilized. Removing and discarding the old problems (programs) such as stress, fear, anxiety, depression, or other phobias does not automatically create a new program. If a person wants to be someone different characteristically, or personality-wise, then the therapist must install a new program that causes the person to feel or act differently. I refer to this new program as the therapy. Some benefits can be derived from the removal of the old problems; but I believe the therapist must, by suggestive therapy, create a new and able program to ensure that the subject does respond either emotionally or physically in a predicted manner.

Two things MUST always be addressed:
1. The events that must be eliminated or created
2. That the person is comfortable participating in the new events and comfortable not doing the things that the person used to do

Without the second, the therapy session may not be successful. Every person goes through the following techniques:
1. Induction
2. Progressive Relaxation

3. Counting Backwards (from 100)
4. Classroom (Deepening Technique)
5. Library
6. Testing (for Depth of Hypnosis)
7. Therapy
8. Returning to Conscious State

1. INDUCTION

Use any induction technique that makes you feel comfortable. Since all induction techniques end up with eye closure, if you have a problem, then just ask the subject to close the eyelids.

2. PROGRESSIVE RELAXATION

When progressive relaxation is properly administered as outlined in this chapter, fifty percent of the subjects enter into a deep state of hypnosis. This will be noticed by the physical appearance of the individual. The individual should appear relaxed with very little, if any, physical movement. Lips are separated, and breathing is slow and regular. However, if you are not satisfied that a deep state of hypnosis has been obtained, then repeat the entire progressive relaxation technique. This is the only deepening technique that can be repeated with success. Should other deepening techniques fail to produce the necessary result, repeating the same will not produce any better results.

3. COUNTING BACKWARDS (from 100)

This technique gives the therapist his first clue as to the depth of hypnosis that has been achieved.

4. CLASSROOM (Deepening Technique)

Two things are accomplished in the classroom:
(1) Development of imagery
(2) Increasing the depth of hypnosis

The classroom combines deepening by design (erasing the letters) and stress (mental disorientation).

5. Library

Age regression to childhood is accomplished. This permits the subject to regress before the initial sensitizing event or events occurred. Removal of the problems (books) for stress, fear, hate, depression, etc. and unwrapping the new books (health and happiness, success and desire) creates a place where the new therapy (programs) can be recorded.

6. Testing (for Depth of Hypnosis)

The number of tests will vary with each individual. Should any test fail to produce the necessary responses, DO NOT REPEAT the same test. Go to a different test. Up to this point in the session, everybody goes through the same procedure. It may be necessary, either before or after the testing, to insert additional deepening techniques such as the elevator, stairway, escalator, or others.

7. Therapy

Up to this point in the sessions, the techniques have been reasonably the same. Here is where the difference takes place, depending on the problems that must be addressed.

8. Returning to Conscious State

Counting up from one to three (or any other number that feels comfortable with the therapist) returns the subject to his conscious state.

Most subjects expect the therapist to do something that causes them to enter into a state of hypnosis. There are two basic induction techniques that I normally use:

1. Taking three deep breaths and exhaling
2. Lowering my hand from above the forehead down to the forehead

Each of these is very effective; however, I really prefer the lowering of the hand down to the forehead.

The deep breathing goes like this:

Get yourself comfortably situated in the chair (or "bed"). Separate your legs, and extend the legs and relax. Arms at your side in a comfortable position. Close your eyelids and keep the eyelids closed. Don't open your eyelids until I ask you to.

And now you take one nice deep breath. Fill your lungs full. Hold it for a moment. Hold it. Hold it. Then slowly exhale and as you exhale, allow your chest muscles and your arms to relax all the way to your fingertips. Now you take another nice, big, deep breath. This time really fill your lungs full. Hold it. Hold it. And now as you exhale, allow your chest muscles and your legs to relax right down to the tip of your toes. Get all the air out. And just one more time, take a big, deep breath. I mean really fill your lungs full, way in. Pull it all in and now hold it. Hold it. Hold it. Now slowly exhale and imagine your body like a balloon and all the air going out and your body deflating, chest relaxing, arms relaxing, stomach muscles and even your legs relaxing. And now you breathe nice and normal, nice and easy. Just take your time and relax.

The other induction which I prefer is to have the person on a bed, a comfortable couch, or a recliner. Make sure the legs are not crossed and the arms are resting on the sides of the body. Standing next to the person, I place my hand about thirty inches above the forehead with the palm down. The hand should be in a position that requires the person to look up over the forehead. In this position, the eyes will automatically become tired, vision blurred, and the eyelids heavy. With the hand in this position, the induction procedure begins as follows:

Look at the palm of my hand. Just by placing my hand in this position to you, I am suggesting relaxation and every time I suggest relaxation, you do relax. Each and every time I suggest relaxation, this causes your eyes to grow tired, causes your eyelids to grow heavy. Now in a moment, I am going to lower my hand down closer to your forehead. As I lower my hand, this causes your eyes to grow more and more tired, causes your eyelids to grow heavy, progressively heavier and heavier. And before my hand touches your forehead, your eyelids do close.

All the time that you are talking, the hand is to remain about thirty inches above the forehead. With the eyes looking up in this position, the eyes are already becoming tired and as the eyes become tired, the eyelids want to close to ease the tired eyes. Now the therapist slowly, very slowly begins to lower the hand down towards the forehead.

Continue as follows:

Now as I lower my hand closer to your forehead, this causes your eyes to grow progressively more and more tired, causes your eyelids to grow heavier and heavier and before my hand touches your forehead, your eyelids do close. Now focus your attention on your arms and relax your arms. Make your arms, from the shoulders down to the elbows, rested and relaxed. Then relax your arms from the elbows down to the wrists.

Relax the back of the hands, even the palms of the
hands. Send this relaxation all the way down to the very
fingertips. Make your arms, from the shoulders all the
way down to the fingertips, totally relaxed and as you
relax your arms, this also causes your eyes to grow even
more tired, causes your eyelids to grow heavy with
relaxation. Eyelids relaxing, relaxing, relaxing and closing
… closing … closed.

With the subject looking up as the hand is lowered, he is
asked to think about relaxing the arms. This creates mental stress
and some confusion. Lowering of the hand is an invasion of the
space, and the only way the person can escape this invasion is to
close the eyelids. Should the eyelids fail to close, then put the hand
over the eyelids, causing the eyelids to close. Then tell the subject
to keep the eyelids closed.

Watch the eyelids and if you see a tendency for the eyelids
to close, just ask the person to close the eyelids. However, if there
is a tendency for the person to fight eye closure, just slow down the
lowering of the hand which, in turn, makes the eyes more tired. In
any event, make sure the eyelids remain closed. Anytime during
the session if the subject opens the eyelids, just ask the person to
close the eyelids and keep the eyelids closed.

If the person refuses to keep the eyelids closed, stop the
session. Explain to the subject that the eyelids must remain closed.
Should the subject continue to open the eyelids, stop the session
and send the person home. Any further attempt will result in failure.

Continue as follows:

Now direct your attention to your eyelids and your
eye muscles, and you relax your eyelids and your eye
muscles. So be aware of what you're doing. Concentrate

or focus your attention on your eyelids and create a feeling in your eyelids and your eye muscles that for you is comfortable, pleasant, peaceful, restful, and relaxing. Hold your direction and attention on your eyelids and eye muscles, and create a feeling of total and complete relaxation just as much as you can. Stay with your eyelids and eye muscles. Really relax those eyelids and eye muscles.

Now you direct your attention to the area around your forehead and your eyebrows. You think about the skin on the forehead, and you make your skin nice and soft. Make the skin smooth and comfortable. If you can, picture and imagine that right on the center of your forehead you have a nice spot ... a dab of creamy, fluffy lotion sitting right on the center of your forehead just above the bridge of your nose. Lotion that you know from past experience is comfortable, lotion that is pleasant, and lotion that penetrates and seeps into the tiny pores of your skin. So imagine this lotion slowly begins to absorb the warmth of your body, and slowly begins to spread and flow across your forehead ... soothing, penetrating, comforting, relaxing all the way down your forehead.

Then imagine this pleasant feeling of comfort slowly trickles and flows from the forehead down, over, and across your temples and down into your cheeks. Now you think about your cheeks and you relax your cheeks. Make your cheek muscles nice and limp and loose and rested and relaxed. Give the cheek muscles the sensation, the symptom, that they want to melt a little bit, trying to let go but still kind of stuck there, and growing progressively more limp, loose, and rested. And you find that each passing moment causes your cheek muscles and your eyelids and eye muscles to relax even more.

So now while your cheek muscles continue to relax even more and more, send some of this relaxation from your cheeks down into your jaw muscles, deep in the jaw muscles. Let the jaw muscles just go limp, loose, and rested. Then, spread this relaxation over to your chin and over to your lips. Now you think about your lips and you relax those lips of yours. Make your lips nice and soft and tender, soothing, comfortable, restful, and relaxing. So you think about your lips ... and let all the muscles in your lips and your mouth muscles relax.

So go ahead and relax everything as much as you can. Relax the jaw muscles, the chin, the cheek muscles, the lips. You see, as you relax all these muscles, your lips have a tendency to part and separate pleasantly and comfortably as this relaxation penetrates even deeper and deeper. And from the forehead, imagine something soothing, something comfortable, something very pleasant slowly flowing and spreading from your forehead up across the top of the head, soothing and caressing the top of the head ... penetrating deep, deep inside ... sending a feeling of comfort deep within.

Imagine this sensation of comfort spreading all the way across the top of the head and the pleasant feeling flows and trickles down the back of your head, soothing and caressing the back of the head. Let this wonderful feeling slowly settle deep into the back of the neck muscles. So you think about all of these areas, and relax each and every one of these areas.

Now imagine that you can experience the sensation, the feeling that this relaxation has a tendency to become loose and the pleasant feeling of relaxation seems to drain down from the top of the head, flow down from the forehead and the eyelids, slowly drain down from the cheeks, seep down from the lips, down through the neck and down to your shoulders, and slowly flow and spread across your shoulders ... touching, soothing, comforting all the shoulder muscles. So now you think about the shoulder muscles. You think about the large and the small muscles in your shoulders, and allow your shoulder muscles to become just totally limp and completely relaxed. Let the shoulder muscles kind of sag and hang a little bit. Just let go. Just let go.

Imagine this wonderful, soothing feeling of relaxation spreads all the way across your shoulders, and now something soothing and comfortable, pleasant and peaceful, flows over your shoulders, down both of your arms. Imagine something so pleasant, so comfortable, so restful and relaxing, flows down both of your arms, not only over the skin but deep, deep inside. Imagine the sensation of relaxation slowly flows downward, downward touching, penetrating, soothing, and caressing all the muscles in both of your arms, resting and relaxing each and every nerve, all the tendons, the fibers ... touching and soothing ... down to your elbows. Now you think about your arms from the elbows to the shoulders, and you let your arms become pleasantly and comfortably and deeply relaxed. As you relax your arms from the shoulders to the elbows, this causes your body to relax from the shoulders down to the hips ... growing more and more relaxed. And now this relaxation continues to flow down past the elbows again over the skin and deep inside your arms ... soothing, comforting all the muscles in both of your arms. Even caressing all of the nerves, tendons, and tissues. Relaxing every cell, every gland, and every fiber. Everything from the elbows all the way down to your wrists.

As you relax your arms from the shoulders down to your wrists, this causes the muscles in your body to relax from the shoulders all the way down to your hips, past your hips all the way down to your toes. Now imagine this relaxation continues to flow down past the wrists. Imagine something so pleasant, so comfortable slowly flowing from the wrists over the back of both of your hands. And a soothing sensation spreads down into the palms of both of your hands. Now all of this relaxation continues to flow down into each and every one of your fingers, causing your arms from the shoulders down to the fingertips to grow more and more relaxed. As you allow your arms to relax from the shoulders past the elbows and down to your finger tips, this causes your whole body to relax from the top of the head down to your shoulders, past your hips, and all the way down to your toes. Each passing moment causes your whole body to relax more and more.

Then imagine this relaxation slowly begins to flow from your shoulders, down your chest, and down your back. Imagine your body being covered, even draped if you like, in the most restful, the most comfortable, the most soothing, the most peaceful sensation you could ever experience ... slowly flowing from the shoulders, down the chest area, penetrating deep in the chest, spreading all the way across the chest, even down the sides of your body. Now from the back of the shoulder, imagine a soothing sensation slowly trickling down through the back muscles, penetrating, resting, relaxing all of the back muscles ... flowing all the way down, down into the lower back.

From the chest area, the sensation of relaxation spreads down and flows into the stomach area. Then all this relaxation continues to flow slowly down into the hips, momentarily stops at the hips but spreads all the way across the hips, penetrating deep, deep in those hips, touching and soothing and caressing all of the muscles, each and every tendon and every nerve and every cell in those hips of yours. You see, I asked you to relax your

body from the top of the head, all the way down to your
hips. Now allow this relaxation to slowly flow down from
the hips, down to the thigh muscles, soothing and
caressing the thigh muscles and then slowly continues to
flow down past the knees, all the way down to your
ankles and into your feet and right to your toes.

You see, it's necessary that you relax your whole
body from the top of the head all the way down to the
toes. Now there's a reason why I asked you to relax
your body. Because in your body, there are all kinds of
human energy. So much energy. But quite a bit of your
energy is locked up, tied up, even knotted up in some of
the cells, the tissues, and the muscles in your body. As
you allow your body to relax, this human energy is
automatically released and untied, set free like tiny
bubbles of energy letting go from your toes.

These bubbles of energy continue to bubble from
your toes, slowly rising up your feet. As these bubbles of
energy rise higher, they bounce against more cells, more
tissues, and more muscles, shaking more bubbles of
energy loose, filling your legs full ... moving, rising,
bouncing bubbles of energy, crowding more bubbles of
energy into your hips and gathering more bubbles of
energy into your stomach area. Now from your
fingertips, bubbles of energy start to let go, and the
bubbles move up into your hands and your arms. These
bubbles of energy ... they too bounce against more
cells, more muscles, more tissues, shaking more bubbles

of energy, filling your arms full of moving, rising, bouncing bubbles of energy. And all these bubbles of energy rise up in your body and gather and converge in your shoulders. Now one by one, the bubbles of energy trickle up the back of your neck, the back of the head to the top of the head. And it's almost like they disappear, but they don't. They just take on a whole new identity.

I'm going to teach you how to redirect this energy so you can fulfill your needs and new desires. So the more you relax, the more energy you have to work with. The more energy you have to work with, the better results you're going to get. All you have to do is just take it easy and relax.

Understand that no time during the course of this session are you going to be unconscious or unaware. So please don't expect this to happen to you. If a car goes by outside and makes a racket, you are going to hear it. My telephone may ring in the other room and if it does, you will hear it. Should I have a need to get up and walk around this room, you will know it. You'll find that nothing bothers you, nothing disturbs you. Whatever you hear just causes you to relax even progressively more and more, feeling more comfortable, more pleasant and more peaceful in your whole mind and your whole body. Your thoughts may drift to another subject. If that happens, don't be concerned about that. That's a normal and natural function of your thinking process.

So if you desire, you can direct your attention back to what I'm talking about. It really doesn't make much difference anymore. You see, your subconscious mind is already open and receptive to everything you and I talk about concerning your needs and your desires.

I'm also satisfied that you recognize you can relax even more than you are now. So in a moment, I'm going to have you count like this: "One hundred ... ninety-nine ... ninety-eight ... ninety-seven ... ninety-six ..." When you start counting, you just whisper and I mean whisper so very softly and slowly, and I mean ever so slowly count backwards. You see, each decreasing number causes you to relax more and more! With each decreasing number, you are relaxing, feeling more comfortable, more pleasant, more peaceful in your whole mind and your whole body.

Now nice and easy, just whisper very softly "one-hundred" and slowly, ever so slowly, count backwards and keep right on counting. Now while you're counting backwards, once again direct your attention to your arms. That's the entire area from the shoulders to the elbows to the wrists to the fingertips. You make those muscles in your arms totally limp and completely relaxed. I mean this time really relax those arms. Make those arms ever so limp and ever so rested and relaxed.

Then direct your attention to your legs and you relax the thigh muscles. You make those thigh muscles ever so limp. Then you spread this relaxation down past your knees, all the way down your legs, down into your ankles and into your toes. You think about your toes way down there. As you allow your arms and your legs to relax, this causes the numbers to lose their importance, already fading away ... disappearing ... going ... going ... and gone. No longer important.

Now I'd like you to picture and imagine that you're standing in a classroom, any kind of a classroom, maybe a schoolroom. It could be one you've been in before or just an imaginary classroom. So picture and imagine you are standing in the classroom and as you look around, you just may see the chairs that the students sit in. They might be a combination desk and chair, an arm chair, or a plain old chair. The students' chairs usually come in rows. Most classrooms have a teacher's desk. Some classrooms have windows. And on the walls, you may find some posters, some pictures, some bulletins, some decorations, maybe some students' work. Then there's this nice blackboard. So picture and imagine that you're standing in a classroom. As you stand in the classroom, look around. You may just see the chairs that the students sit in, possibly a teacher's desk, something on the walls, and the blackboard.

Should the subject or patient be over 50 years old, you may refer to the writing board as a blackboard. However, if the subject is under 50, you may address the board as a white board or a chalkboard. Use your discretion, depending on the age and the experience of each individual. Repeat the nature of the board as often as you can. The classroom is where you begin to create imagery. The more often the board is repeated, the more distinct the imagery becomes. The imagery that you build in the classroom is then more fully utilized in the library.

Continue as follows:

When the picture of the blackboard is reasonably clear in your mind, nod your head YES. Walk over to the blackboard. You stand about a foot, maybe a foot and a half, away from the blackboard. Face the blackboard and you look at the blackboard. Standing so close to the blackboard, facing the blackboard, looking at the blackboard, chances are all you can see is this blackboard. So while you're standing facing the blackboard, looking at the blackboard, allow your eyes to drift down to the bottom of the blackboard, and there's a ledge.

On the ledge is a piece of chalk and an eraser. With one hand, you pick up the chalk and with the other, you pick up the eraser. Now you should be standing, facing the blackboard, holding the chalk in one hand and the eraser in the other hand. When you have the chalk in one hand and the eraser in the other, nod your head YES so I know you have the chalk in one hand and the eraser in the other. I said, "Pick up the chalk," but for you it may be a marker or some other writing tool. Whatever it is, a marker or something else, I am going to call this writing instrument ... chalk.

Everything is quiet and pleasant and peaceful. With each passing moment, you'll find that the picture of this blackboard in the classroom grows clearer and clearer and more distinct as though somebody turned on some lights. Now with the chalk you have in one hand, slowly and very carefully write the letter A on the blackboard. Take your time, slow and easy. We're in no hurry. When you have the letter A on the blackboard, with the eraser you have in the other hand, slowly and so very carefully erase the letter A from the blackboard. When the letter A has been erased from the blackboard, nod your head YES that you have erased the letter A from the blackboard.

It is important that you be aware of all the movements of the person being hypnotized. Don't be afraid to ask the person if he has completed the task that you request.

Continue as follows:

With the chalk you still have in one hand, slowly and carefully draw the letter B on the blackboard. The letter B is a nice letter. The letter B has a lot of twists and some loops and some turns. When you still have the letter B on the blackboard, with the eraser again, slowly, nicely, and easily erase the letter B from the blackboard. When the letter B has been erased from the blackboard, nod your head YES that you have erased the letter B from the blackboard.

With the chalk you still have in one hand, slowly and carefully write the letter C on the blackboard. The letter C is an easy letter to write. When you have the letter C on the blackboard, then with the eraser you still have in one hand, slowly and carefully erase the letter C from the blackboard. Take your time. And when the letter C has been erased from the blackboard, nod your head YES that you have erased the letter C from the blackboard.

Now in a moment, I'm going to have you continue with the rest of the alphabet. When I ask you to start, I want you to start with the letter D. But please don't start until I ask you to. You see, I'm going to have you write the letter D very slowly and very carefully, and then I'm going to have you erase the letter D slowly and carefully. Then I'm going to ask you to continue slowly writing and erasing the letters of the alphabet, and you'll find that each movement of the eraser causes you to relax progressively more and more. With each movement of the eraser, you are relaxing, feeling more comfortable, more pleasant, more peaceful in your mind and body. Now you may start with the letter D. Slowly and carefully, write the letter D and when the letter D is on the blackboard, nice and easy with the eraser, carefully erase the letter D from the blackboard. Then you continue slowly writing and erasing the letters of the alphabet while I talk to you ...

You might remember when you first became acquainted with the letters of the alphabet, some of the letters were simple, other letters were difficult, and there were some letters that were confusing. The easy letters could have been the O, the S, the X, or the T. But there were the P and the Q kind of twisted backwards. You might have had a problem with the D and the B, the M and the N, or the U, the V, and the W. Then when you decided to recite the alphabet, there was a time when you got to a certain letter in the alphabet and you couldn't remember the next succeeding letter. The harder you tried, the more difficult it became so you decided to go back to A and B and C, hoping to pick one you couldn't remember. Now as you continue to erase, go ahead and erase away all the remaining letters of the alphabet, no more important, let them fade away ... disappearing ... going ... going ... and gone.

When you start with the above words, "You might remember when you first became acquainted ...," speak a little faster than usual. This is the time to start some mental confusion. While the person is writing and erasing the letters of the alphabet beginning with "D," you keep talking about the other letters so rapidly, the person is not able to think about what he is supposed to be writing and erasing. So on his own, he just quits writing and erasing. This mental confusion drops the subject into a deeper state of hypnosis.

Continue as follows:

Now you put the chalk and eraser back on the ledge. Then look around in this classroom. As you look around in the classroom, you'll find there is a closed door in this classroom and this door leads from the

classroom. So look around this classroom. When you
recognize the closed door, nod your head YES.

If you believe at this point the patient is not in a deep enough
state of hypnosis, you would now take the patient from the
classroom into a hallway that leads to an elevator. This deepening
technique is covered in Chapter 8.

Continue as follows:

Now the door you're looking at leads to a library.
You know what a library looks like. A library has many,
many bookshelves, bookshelves in so many, many rows.
On these bookshelves are so many, many books. A
library is a nice place, a pleasant place, a nice place to
think.

Walk over to the library door, open the library door,
step into the library, and then close the library door
behind you. Now look around in this library and when
you see the bookshelves in rows, just nod your head YES
that you see the bookshelves in rows.

When the subject nods his head "yes" that the bookshelves
are visible, feel good; for the subject will see everything else you
say is in the library.

Continue as follows:

In a moment, I am going to ask you to select any
aisle in this library and I'm going to ask you to walk to
that aisle and stand between two bookshelves and look
down the aisle. As you look down the aisle, you will find

the books on the right side of this aisle are nice books, good books, books that have been read and used. On the other side of the aisle, the books are not so good.

So select any aisle and walk to that aisle, stand between the bookshelves and look down the aisle. The books on the right side are nice books, good books, books that have been read and used. Books on the other side are not so good. So when you are standing between the bookshelves and looking down the aisle, nod your head YES that you are standing between the bookshelves.

The hypnotist should always refer to the right side of the aisle as the good side, nice side, pleasant side, or right side. There is no left side or bad side. The other side is called the "not-so-good side," "other side," or "problem side."

Continue as follows:

As you look down the aisle, all of these books are about you. Everything that you did in your entire lifetime is recorded in the books as you look down the aisle. Not only everything you did, but also everything that you thought about is also recorded in these books as you look down the aisle. All of your past emotions, feelings and symptoms, fantasies and dreams are also recorded and these books do contain everything that you have read, what you heard, and what you saw in your entire lifetime.

The books on the right side, the nice books, they hold your pleasant experiences, your wonderful thoughts, your good emotions and feelings, symptoms, fantasies, even dreams. So the nice books on the right side, they hold and contain and have recorded all the nice things you ever did in your whole lifetime, your beautiful thoughts that you had in your whole lifetime, the pleasant feelings and emotions and your nice dreams. The books on the other side hold and contain those that, for you, haven't been so nice.

The books closest to you hold and contain your most <u>recent</u> experiences. That's what you did today, yesterday, and the day before. Not only your most <u>recent</u> experiences, but also your most <u>recent</u> thoughts. Even your most <u>recent</u> feelings and emotions, your most <u>recent</u> symptoms, fantasies, and dreams are recorded in the books closest to you. The most <u>recent</u> things you saw and what you read and the things you heard are also recorded in the books nearest you.

The books farther down the aisle are about you when you were <u>younger and smaller</u>. The books farther down the aisle have recorded and do contain the things you did when you were <u>younger and smaller</u>. The thoughts you had when you were <u>younger and smaller</u> are also contained in the books farther down the aisle. Your symptoms, feelings, and emotions that you had when you were <u>younger</u> are also contained in the books farther down the aisle. The books farther down the aisle also contain the things you heard what you saw and read when you were <u>younger and smaller</u>.

The books on the far end of this aisle are about you when you were just a baby. So these books on the far end of this aisle contain what you did when you were a baby and what you thought about when you were a baby. All of your feelings and emotions that you experienced when you were a baby are contained in the books at the far end.

All of these books that you see down the aisle have pictures. Pictures of everything that you did in your entire lifetime. And I am not going to ask you what's in any of your books.

Turn and look at the books on the right side, the nice side. Keep your eyes on the books on the right side, the nice books. Now slowly, very slowly, walk down the aisle. If you like, touch the books as you go by.

Walk about halfway down the aisle and stop. When you get about halfway down the aisle, reach up on the right side. Take a book off the shelf. Hold this book in your hands. You see the book you're holding now is about you when you were younger and smaller. When you have this book in your hands, nod your head YES that you have this book in your hand.

(The subject nods his head.)

This book has pictures, pleasant pictures of some nice things you did when you were younger and smaller. Open this book to a picture of you doing something when you were younger and smaller. If you like or need, turn the pages. When you see a picture of you doing something when you were younger, just nod your head YES.

(The subject nods his head.)

That's fine. Now close the book and put the book back on the shelf on the right side.

> If after a short time the subject doesn't nod "yes," just ask the person to close the book and return the book back to the shelf on the right side. Don't be concerned if the person doesn't see a picture. The pictures are on the other side, the not-so-good side. Just continue with the session.

Continue as follows:

Still keeping your eyes on the right side, the nice side, slowly, very slowly, walk down the aisle. Touch and feel the books as you go by. Walk all the way down to the end of the bookshelf and stop. Then take one small step backward.

Now reach up on the right side and take another book off the shelf. Hold this book in your hands. When you have this book in your hands, then nod your head YES so I know that you have this book in your hands.

(The subject nods his head.)

This book is about you when you were just a baby. This book has pleasant pictures of the lovely things you did when you were just a baby. So give this book a hug, a hug and a squeeze to your chest. It's a treasured book of beautiful experiences and wonderful pictures of the nice things you did when you were just a baby.

Open this book to a picture about you doing something pleasant when you were just a baby. If you like and need, turn the pages and when you see a picture of you doing something when you were just a baby, just nod your head YES that you see the picture.

(The subject nods his head.)

Close the book and put the book back on the shelf on the right side.

Age regression has just been accomplished. The patient was taken back from the present to the time when the patient was a baby. Using this technique, the therapist need not be concerned about taking the person back to the initial sensitizing event. Taking the person back to childhood or to the time that the patient was a baby, in all likelihood, was before the initial sensitizing event. With this technique, you never run into a traumatic event or abreaction.

Continue as follows:

Now turn and look at the books on the other side. These books are not-so-nice. Some of the books, only some of the books, are problem books. You see, every problem that you ever had in your whole lifetime has its own book. Every problem has its own title. And in that problem book are all of your experiences as they relate to that particular problem. That's a lifetime of experiences which are related to that particular problem. Also recorded in that problem book are all of the thoughts you had in your whole lifetime concerning that problem, together with all of your emotions, feelings, your symptoms, your fantasies, and your dreams that relate to that problem in that problem book.

On the not-so-nice side, the other side, the problem side, you've got a book up there that has a title Stress, S-T-R-E-S-S. So look around on the not-so-nice side, the problem side, and when you recognize your Stress problem book, reach up and take your stress problem off the shelf. When you have this stress problem in your hands, nod your head YES.

(The subject nods his head.)

When the book is on the shelf, it is called a *Stress* problem book or *Weight* problem book or *Drug* problem book or whatever the name should be. When the book is taken off the shelf, you make a conversion. Now it is called a "stress problem," "weight problem," or whatever name of the problem you are treating. On the shelf it is a book; but once in the subject's hands, it is a problem.

Continue as follows:

Hold the stress problem in your hands and understand what you're holding. You're holding in your hands every past stressful experience you ever had in your whole lifetime. You're holding in your hands every past stressful thought and all of your past stressful emotions and feelings, even your past stressful dreams. You are also holding in your hands everything that you saw, heard, and read about that, for you, was stressful.

Some of these have a tendency to creep into today's and tomorrow's conduct, and mess up today's and the future's pleasures. What you are really holding in your hands are ashes of yesterday's experiences, ashes of yesterday's thoughts, ashes of yesterday's emotions and feelings as they relate to stress, no longer important to you in the light of today's circumstances.

On the aisle you're standing in, there is a container. So look around on the floor of this aisle and find the container. When you recognize the container on the floor of this aisle, you take your stress problem to the container and you throw your stress problem into that container. Just get rid of your stress problem, no longer important for you. When your stress problem is in the container, nod your head YES that you have discarded your stress problem.

(The subject nods his head.)

As you conduct the interview with the persons, take notes as to their expressions so that you can make a list of the problem books. Use their language for the titles. Some titles may be *Fear, Anxiety, Guilt, Shame, Smoking, Drugs, Alcohol*, etc. Some titles may be names of persons who have given them problems. In the case of names, explain that you are not eliminating the person, but only the not-so-nice experiences, thoughts, or feelings that have been created by that person.

Every problem has its own book. The first book is always the *Stress* book and the last book at the first session is the *I-Can't* book and/or *Excuses* book. In most cases, do not handle more than four problems at the same session. In subsequent sessions, throw some of the other problems into the container. Do not describe the container. Let the individual create his own container's identity.

Continue as follows:

Now go back to the problem side, the not-so-nice side, that's the other side over there. You have another problem over there. You have a book that has a title, I-Can't.

You see every I-Can't that you ever used, every I-Can't that you ever thought about, every I-can't that you ever created was put into your I-Can't problem book, sentence after sentence, page after page, chapter after chapter. You've got a book full of I-Can'ts.

When you recognize your I-Can't problem book, take your I-Can't problem off the shelf and hold this I-Can't problem in your hands. Now understand what you're really holding. What you're holding in your hands are your self-imposed limitations, your self-imposed restrictions, your self-imposed inhibitions. You see, you surrendered control over some of the things you do, some of the things you think about and how you feel. You take your I-Can't problem over to that container but don't throw the I-Can't problem in the container.

You sit on the floor next to the container and put your I-Can't problem in your lap. Open up the cover and tear out the first page. Tear the first page in small pieces. Throw the pieces into the container. And then you proceed to tear out each and every one of your I-Can'ts. Tear all of your I-Can'ts in small pieces and throw all of the pieces into the container.

As you tear up your I-Can'ts, this causes you to free
yourself and your subconscious mind of each and every
one of your limitations, all your restrictions, and every
one of your inhibitions. As you tear up your I-Can'ts,
this causes you to take back total and complete control
over everything you do, everything that you think
about, and especially how you feel. So, feel good about
tearing up your I-Can'ts. When all of your I-Can'ts have
been torn up and thrown into the container, toss the
cover into the container.

When the cover's in the container, go back to the not-
so-nice side, the problem side. You may have some more
problems up there. Understand that every problem that
you've had in your whole lifetime has its own book, and
every problem has its own title. In that problem book are all
of your experiences as they relate to that particular
problem, and all your thoughts, emotions and feelings,
fantasies and dreams as it concerns that particular problem.
So look around. You may find other problems up there.

So understand that for every problem that you had in
your lifetime, there is a book, and the book has a title of
your problem ... so be selective and look around ... and
when you recognize your problems, take your problems
off the shelf and throw your problems into the container.

Should you need another container, look around.
There's another container that's available. You might even
be surprised that this container that you have now might

even grow for you. So feel free. Take your problems off
the shelf. Throw your problems into the container.

I'll give you a few moments to look around. Look for
your problems and take your problems off the shelf. Throw
your problems into the container ... and think, "Hey, it's
about time I got rid of that problem!" ... so take your
time. Be selective. Be honest with yourself. Feel good
about what you're doing. You see, you're disposing of the
old problems, yesterday's problems, yesterday's thoughts,
yesterday's experiences, emotions, yesterday's feelings.
So go ahead and get rid of your past problems.

When you have finished throwing away your past
problems, just nod your head YES, then we can continue.
But take your time and clean house, that is, get rid of
your unwanted problems.

(The therapist pauses and allows the subject to get rid of the
problems.) (The subject nods his head.)

Now I'll tell you what to do. You stand back, away
from the container or containers, whatever the case may
be. Watch the containers slide and glide away from you.
A door in the library opens and right through the
doorway go the containers, carrying all of the problems
you decided to dispose of. When the containers and the
problems have gone right through the doorway, the door
automatically closes and you may hear the door lock
tight. When the door is closed, just nod your head YES,
so I know the door is closed.

(The subject nods his head.)

When the door is locked nice and tight, you go back
to the right side, the first side, nice side. On the bottom
shelf are the books that are wrapped up. When you
recognize the wrapped books, nod your head YES that
you see the wrapped up books.

(The subject nods his head.)

Reach down and pick up a book that is wrapped up
and hold this book in your hands, and understand that
this book you're holding also has a title. The title of this
book is Health and Happiness. When you have the
Health and Happiness book in your hands, just nod your
head YES that you have your Health and Happiness book
in your hands.

(The subject nods his head.)

Unwrap your Health and Happiness book and when
your Health and Happiness book is unwrapped, you
place that Health and Happiness book on the right side,
a position that's important because for you this is a very,
very important book.

Repetition is the basis upon which imagery is created and
maintained. So repeat the name of the books as often as you can.
This may sound strange or even ridiculous, but I find I get much
better results with the repetitions. Should you use words that have
multiple meanings, the conscious mind is automatically elevated
to make the interpretation.

Continue as follows:

When you have your Health and Happiness book on
the shelf, then reach down and pick another wrapped book.

This book also has a title. The title of this book is Success. Unwrap the Success book, then place your Success book on the shelf on the right side, close to the Health and Happiness book. Now you should have two books on the shelf, Health and Happiness and Success, two very important books in your library, your memory bank.

When your Success book is on the shelf, then reach down one more time and pick up another book that is wrapped up. When you have this book in your hands, just nod your head YES so I know that you have this book. (The subject nods his head.)

Give this book a big hug and a squeeze, for this is a very important book. The title of this book is Desires. Every desire that you have ever had in your whole life for health and happiness and success is in this book. Every desire, whether it is physical desire, spiritual desire, or material desire for health and happiness and success, is in this Desires book.

Notice how often certain words are repeated. This may seem somewhat redundant, but understand that the more often the word is repeated, the more distinct the image appears. Whatever is important should be repeated as often as necessary to achieve the best images.

Unwrap your Desires book and put your Desires book up on the shelf close to the other two books. Now you should have three books on the shelf: Health and Happiness, Success, and Desires. When your Desires

book is up on the shelf, walk back up the aisle to the
point where you first entered this aisle and close by is a
nice, comfortable easy chair, a recliner, in your library.
You go sit down in your comfortable easy chair in the
library and take it easy.

Now think about what you just did. You went back
in time to when you were a child. Then you went on the
other side, the not-so-nice side, the problem side and you
found some of your past problems. You took your past
problems off the shelf. You threw your past problems in a
container and you saw the container leave with all of the
past problems.

So what you did was mind surgery. You see, a
surgeon may open up the area around a person's
stomach and take out an appendix that has given a
person some difficulty. Once the appendix has been
removed and cast aside, the appendix can't bother the
person anymore. Or a dentist may extract a troublesome
tooth. Once a tooth has been extracted and cast aside,
that tooth won't bother that person anymore.

You found some problems that have been bothering
you over a period of time. You took your problems off
the shelf. You threw your problems in the container and
now they're gone. Since they're gone, they can't bother
you anymore, not today, not tomorrow, not ever. So feel
good about what you did. You got rid of all of your past
problems that you decided to get rid of.

Now it is the time for the testing of the depth of hypnosis. Therapy should not be conducted unless the therapist is satisfied by the test that the subject is in a state of deep hypnosis; that is, when the suggestion is done in a state of deep hypnosis, the subject's reaction and response will be that the suggestion is true. Understand, unless rejected, that the suggestions are true.

When you want the subject to do something like relaxing the legs or any part of the legs, give the person time to accomplish this task. For example, "Relax your thigh muscles, make your thigh muscles limp and rested ... relax your legs from the knees down to the ankles ... just focus your attention on the leg muscles and relax the leg muscles..." Nothing exists in the patient's body until you create it. And how do you create it? You make the suggestion. You make the suggestion and let the patient create the condition. And then it happens. You see, the hypnotist has no control over the body. The body responds to the patient's thoughts. But your thoughts and your suggestions and your ideas, as hypnotist, cause the individual to think along the lines that you're suggesting.

So in a state of hypnosis when you do the testing, the individual patient should not be given the opportunity to form any individual thoughts. As long as you keep talking, the patient must respond.

Normally, the test will proceed by an indirect route. If you want the leg to become heavy so the subject can't lift it, don't start at the leg. If you want the arm to become totally limp and can't be lifted, don't start at the arm.

You may want to start with something like this:

Now you sit in that comfortable chair and just let yourself relax. Let your whole body relax. Why don't you relax your legs? That's the thigh muscles, past your knees, down to the ankles, and down to the toes. Let your legs relax pleasantly and comfortably. Relax your arms, shoulders, all the tissues down to the elbows and to the fingertips. Let your arms go limp. If you like, you can even relax your stomach muscles and your chest. Let those shoulders relax. You can relax your eyelids if you like, and let your cheek muscles and your lips relax.

And as you allow your body to relax, you may experience that your left leg seems to relax more than the rest of your body. Why, the left leg may seem to be growing pleasantly relaxed, comfortably relaxed, maybe a little bit numb, a little bit useless. That's OK.

You may even recognize the shoe on the end of your foot, and the shoe may get heavier and heavier, and the leg relaxes more and more. The shoe may even feel like a boot, like a heavy boot, like a heavy lead boot. Like an anchor on the end of the leg. Like an anchor that's chained down to the floor. And so heavy is the anchor and is so relaxed is your leg that you can't even pick up your left leg.

As you think about lifting your left leg, your very thoughts cause your left leg to grow progressively numb and useless, cause the anchor to grow heavy, so very heavy. So you think about that left leg of yours and you direct your attention to your left leg and you think about that left leg and you try to pick your left leg up and you find you can't even budge it. Won't even move. Anchor's too heavy. Leg is totally numb and useless.

So go ahead and think about that left leg. Direct your attention to that leg. So be aware of what you're doing and you find you can't lift it. It won't even budge. Just totally limp and useless. So you think about the left leg and you try to pick it up, but you can't.

Now I'm going to pick up your left arm nice and easy by the elbow and the wrist, and put the palm of your hand right on your thigh. And your hand, acting like a sponge now, begins to absorb all the numbness, that heaviness, the useless feeling from your whole leg, sucked into the tiny little hand, and the hand becoming progressively more numb and useless and heavy with relaxation, leg growing perfectly normal, wonderful and pleasant.

So I am going to pick up that arm nice and easy and gently put that hand on your neck and gently stroke your hand and as I do so, this causes the numbness to flow from your hand into your neck. Penetrating deeper and deeper, spreading down into your neck, down into your throat, down into the vocal chords. Numbness spreads into your jaw muscles, your chin, and up into your lips. Seeps between the lips, down into the mouth, down into the tongue, and all the way down into your throat into your vocal chords, causing the vocal chords to become totally numb and completely useless. So useless you can't speak one word.

I'm going to ask you some questions and you know all the answers to my questions, <u>but as you think about the answers, the very thoughts cause</u> cotton balls to form in your throat, cause your tongue to become numb and useless and cause your lips to turn to wax. Thick, heavy wax so you can't speak even one word. Why, you can't even tell me your first name.

Now you think about that and you know your first name. You try to tell me your first name, but you can't talk. Nothing moves. Totally numb and completely useless ... why, you can't even tell me what city you live in. Now you know what city you live in, so you think about the city and you find you can't speak one word. Not one. Why, you can't even tell what day of the week it is. Now you think about that. You can't speak one word. Not one word at all.

Now I'm going to place my hand on your forehead nice and easy and as I do so, this causes the numbness and useless feeling to leave your neck, your throat and vocal chords, your lips, your tongue. The numb and useless feeling leaves your whole body.

And now the hypnotist gently places his hand on the subject's forehead and keeps the hand right on the forehead.

Continue as follows:

You can speak clearly and distinctly. As a matter of fact, you speak better than you did before, diction excellent, enunciation perfect. Hey, the words just seem to flow right out ... nice and easy. So go ahead, tell me your first name. That's fine. And where do you live? That's fine. What day of the week is it? See, you speak clearly and distinctly and that's all right.

When doing the testing, the therapist must speak just a little faster. It is not necessary to hurry the words but continue to talk. You might even prepare an advanced script for the testing and then the script can be read without too much hesitation or confusion. Hesitation or delay in speaking allows the subject to entertain his own thoughts and this is what must be avoided.

By transferring the numbness from the thigh to the hand, this same transference can follow by touching any part of the body that has some pain or discomfort. With the suggestion that as the palm of the hand touches the area of the pain, this touching causes the pain to dissipate and go away. So understand that the anesthesia created in the thigh can be moved to any part of the body by suggestion.

In the event that the patient (subject) is to undergo a surgical procedure, the following suggestions may also be added: "As the area is touched by a surgeon, physician, nurse, or attendant with a gloved hand, instrument, linen material, fluid, or any material, this causes the area touched to grow progressively more and more numb. Each subsequent touch causes the numbness to penetrate deeper and deeper within the area and spread further and further."

When you are satisfied that the patient is in a deep state of hypnosis, begin the suggestive therapy.

Continue as follows:

So you sit in that comfortable chair and you think, "If I could be the person I would like to be, that is personality-wise or characteristically, who would I be? And if I could do the things I would like to do, what would I do? If I could discard, put away, eliminate from my life the things I would like to get rid of, what would I change? And if I could feel like I would like to feel under any set of conditions or circumstances, how would I feel?"

So imagine that as you sit in the comfortable chair, you made a transition and now you are the person you would like to be and you do the things you would like to do and you never do the things you don't like to do and you feel like you would like to feel under any set of circumstances and conditions. Think about it.

Imagine that you could extend your hands and arms up towards the ceiling and roof without doing any damage, and your hands and arms extend up into the sky, farther than you can even see and by doing so, you are able to grasp the future and pull the future down over you and into you. By doing so, you just became the person that you would like to be personality-wise, characteristically.

Now you do the things that you like to do and you no longer do those things that you have no need or desire to do and now you feel like you desire to feel in any set of circumstances and conditions. Think about that. You just made a transition and now you are the person that you would like to be. No longer are you the person you used to be. You have just made the change.

Since everything you do in life is preceded by a thought and all of your emotions, feelings, and symptoms are also preceded by a thought, now you must tell your brain who you are (characteristically), what you do, and what you don't do and how you feel doing the things that you like to do and how you feel not doing the things that you have discarded.

You are now ready for your suggestive therapy.

Your suggestive therapy must follow a particular and prescribed pattern. First of all, the word <u>will</u> should never be used in your suggestive therapy. The word <u>will</u> means something is going to happen in the future, but you only function now in the present time. All your suggestions must be in the present tense. You see, for you everything begins now and continues into the future.

Two things you're going to think about. One is the event you wish to create or the event you wish to eliminate. The second is how you feel doing the things you like to do and how you feel not doing the things you have no desire to do. The second is equally as important as the first.

So imagine that you're sitting in that comfortable chair in your library and you just became that kind of person and if I were to ask you, "Well, who are you now? Not who you used to be," I want to know what transition you made and who you are now.

I'd expect you to say to me, "Oh, you want to know who I am now?" I'd say, YES. I'd expect you to say to me, "Well, first of all, I am the most relaxed person you could ever possibly meet. I'm so relaxed and so comfortable that nothing bothers me. Nobody, nobody disturbs me, not today, not tomorrow, not ever. You see,

I'm in total control of everything I ever do, whatever I think about and how I feel, and I sure love who I am." So if you want to be that kind of person, then you have to tell yourself, "I am."

You see, what happens, you put the messages into that brain for storage. Then at a given time or place, or at your request, these messages, these instructions are processed. And yes, you do become the person you think you are and you do the things that you say you do and you do feel the way you say you feel under any set of circumstances or any place or conditions. Then I'd expect you to say to me, besides being such a nice, relaxed person, "I'm a very compassionate person. I'm a lovable person. I'm an interesting person. I'm even a happy, joyful person."

So if you want to be that kind of person, tell yourself, "I am." Then you can continue and say, "I'm a competent person, capable beyond all expectations. That's me ... I'm successful in everything I do. Everything I do, I do with comfort and with complete success. You see, I do things right the first time, on time, never delayed. I'm also an honest, trustworthy person, I am a completely reliable person."

So, understand if you want to be a particular kind of person, who you want to be characteristically, there are no limitations on what you can cause to be created. But you must tell yourself, "That's who I am." Because if you think you are, the subconscious mind says, "Hey brain, guess who this person thinks this person is? We have to create the condition, the set of circumstances. We must make this person in the image of his thoughts."

You see, everything is preceded by a thought. If you do not have the thought, the brain cannot process anything. Then I expect you to go on and tell me what you do. "I am the best in what I do. None better. I'm the best at my work. I'm the best socially. I'm the best with my family." So if you want to do something, you must tell yourself, "I do."

But the key is to be specific and detailed, what you do and how you feel.

Up to this point in the session, we have only treated the subject's symptoms and emotions, so now we must proceed to handle the changes in the activities, the things the person participates in. For this session, we will assume the person would like to stop smoking cigarettes.

Continue as follows:

Understand that each day you live, you do add more and more pages and books to your memory bank, your library. Select only those thoughts and events that meet your new needs and desires. You are in charge. You are the only one who can get into your memory bank, your library.

The smoking book held all of those thoughts, events, and impressions that you used to consider beneficial about smoking. All those impressions and thoughts implied that smoking a cigarette did something good for

you, but you now know that smoking is dangerous to
your health, that it does make you ill and it does break
down your immune system. Now you have no need or
desire to smoke. All of your past needs and desires to
smoke have gone. You have removed them.

Each and every one of your excuses for smoking is
also gone. You found the Excuse book. You reached up on
the shelf, took the book off the shelf, and destroyed each
and every one of the excuses that have caused you to
continue taking the poison in white paper. You, all by
yourself, destroyed each and every excuse. Now you have
no excuse to take the poison wrapped in white paper.

One of your excuses that caused you to continue to
smoke was that you would gain weight if you stopped.
That excuse is now gone with each and every other excuse.
Now that you have stopped smoking, there is no need to
eat to excess. You do eat only such amount of food that is
necessary to sustain you in your daily activities.

You never missed taking poison before, and now you
feel perfectly comfortable and satisfied in mind and body
without the poison wrapped in white paper that you used
to call cigarettes. They are no longer cigarettes. They
are poison wrapped in white paper.

Over the years you have been telling yourself that
you can't quit smoking. Each time you repeated "I-
can't," you compounded the suggestion that you
couldn't quit smoking. Your subconscious mind wouldn't

let you quit. You didn't have a choice. Your subconscious mind had to follow your previous instructions that you couldn't quit and it wouldn't let you stop taking the poison in white paper. These instructions to your subconscious mind were removed by you when you got rid of the books that held all of your previous instructions. You are finally free. Now you can do anything you have a desire and a need to do.

You came here today because of your new needs and desires. The most important thing on your mind today is to leave the poison alone. No longer are these old instructions of "I-Can't" going to control your actions. Now you can do anything you have a need or desire to do. You are in charge of all of your actions and conduct. No longer are you a slave to cigarettes, the poison wrapped in white paper. You never in the past had a desire for poison and now you have no need or desire for any kind of poison, no matter how it is packaged, especially the poison in white paper.

Every page in every book in this library and each and every book that you add to this library from today, I want to contain good and positive thoughts. You are in control of what is put into your library, memory bank. Make these thoughts good ones, pleasant ones, comforting and satisfying ones. Life can be happy, wonderful, and worthwhile. Each thought that you plant causes your body to respond, so I want you to think of those things that are pleasant and satisfying, and your body then will respond in a pleasant and satisfying manner.

Remember that the thought comes first and the body responds. The thought is the energy, the impulse, the instruction to the brain to start in motion the conduct you wish to follow. Upon receiving this impulse, the brain causes the nerves to transmit the messages to that portion or part of your body to be affected. You are now in charge of your body. So create the messages and those impulses that meet with your new needs and desires.

By removing those books that contained all of the old instructions, you cleared your brain of your old behavioral patterns and are now ready for the new instructions. No one else can enter your library. No one can put any books there. You are now in charge. Recognize that you have removed all of your old problems and are now ready to recite to your subconscious mind the new instructions contained in your new Health and Happiness and Success books. The instructions in these good books state that from this moment and for the rest of your life you have no need for cigarettes, poison in white paper. You have no need now, no desires now, and will have no need and desire for the rest of your life.

The label on that package of cigarettes says that "Smoking is dangerous to your health," not that it might be dangerous, but that it is dangerous to your health. It is poison wrapped in white paper, the most dangerous kind. The effect is not immediate. It sneaks up over the years and before you realize it, your health is gone forever. When you do want to quit smoking? While you are still healthy or when it's too late? Certainly when you are healthy.

Congratulate yourself, give yourself credit for making a decision to stay healthy, and enjoy the fruits of your years of labor. These new instructions are now locked up in your brain, your memory bank, and readily available to your subconscious mind to read. These instructions stand out like a red flag, always present.

Over the years, you were aware of the label of poison on various products such as acids, lye, Drain-o, and other household products. I'm sure you never had a craving for sulfuric or muriatic acids or lye or any product that carried a label signifying a skull and crossbones. You never said to yourself, "I'm dying for a drink of poison." You were perfectly content, satisfied, and comfortable in mind and body without any poison, no matter how it was packaged.

The very thought of taking poison is unacceptable to you. As a matter of fact, it is repulsive in every respect to your mind and body as a whole. Everything in your life that you know causes you harm has always been and still is unacceptable and repulsive to you. Now you recognize that cigarettes are dangerous to your health. Your subconscious mind is being instructed to reject the use of poison wrapped in white paper. They are no longer cigarettes in your mind but poison wrapped in white paper. Cigarettes are repulsive to you in your mind and body. They are dangerous to your health.

Your subconscious mind is now being instructed that from this moment on and for the rest of your life, cigarettes are repulsive. Your subconscious mind is further instructed to do everything in its power never to permit you to waver from your desire to keep your body healthy in every respect. You have too much to live for to take poison and destroy your future. Each and every time that you just think about putting a cigarette in your mouth with the intention of smoking the cigarette, your very thoughts cause every cell in your body to literally scream, "NO, NO, DON'T PUT THAT CIGARETTE IN THIS BODY."

Each and every thought about smoking causes the stomach muscles to tighten up, causing the stomach to grow nauseated and completely upset. Each subsequent thought about smoking a cigarette causes you to become more and more frustrated and upset.

And so, too, each and every thought and word rejecting smoking cigarettes causes you to feel comfortable, relaxed, and very pleasant just like you drank the most soothing, satisfying, and refreshing liquid. Each subsequent time that you reject smoking cigarettes causes you to feel progressively more and more comfortable.

Each and every time you think or speak words such as, "I don't smoke anymore," or, "'I am a non-smoker," or, "I refuse to put cigarettes in my body," or any such rejections of cigarettes cause you to feel progressively more relaxed and comfortable.

At this time, additional phrases may be added such as, "Cigarette smoke tastes like sulfur or burning rubber," "Cigarette smoke is absolutely repulsive," "Cigarette smoke tastes like … *[Name something the person cannot tolerate]*."

Continue as follows:

When you unwrapped your Health and Happiness, Success, and Desires books, you made three commitments. You made a commitment that whatever you do today and every day, you do these things because what you do causes you to feel healthy and happy. Your Health and Happiness book contains a statement that says, "Subconscious mind, never allow me or cause me to do anything that causes me to feel unhappy and causes me to be unhealthy."

Your Success book says you are now successful in everything you do. And whatever you do, you do right the first time and on time, no delays. You made a commitment when you unwrapped your Desires book to fulfill each and every one of your desires, whether they are physical, spiritual, or material, for health and happiness and success.

The unwrapping of the *Health and Happiness* and *Success* books is a very simple, logical, and acceptable means of implanting within the subject's subconscious mind his needs and desires. During the interview, the subject will confidently reveal his desires to the hypnotist. The hypnotist, by suggestion, causes the hidden goals to emerge with the new book and be imprinted on the memory bank.

Taking the wrapping from the books is tantamount to freeing the potential within the subject. Many subjects or patients will state that a burden has been removed from their shoulders, and a noticeable air of freedom will appear in their conduct.

Continue as follows:

I am going to count from one to three and at the count of three, your eyelids do open, you are alert and in your conscious state of awareness, feeling wonderful and relaxed. One ... two ... and three. Eyelids open, fully alert, and feeling comfortable and relaxed.

Let the subject take credit for finding and removing the books from the shelves, destroying and throwing the books into the container. By being reassured that he has done the work, he gains a certain amount of self-respect and confidence. It is he, after all, who is responsible for his own results.

The brain is the memory bank, the library that retains all of the thoughts, impulses, impressions, and events from the beginning of time. The subconscious mind merely seeks out that which it, in most cases, has caused to be stored without the benefit of the analytical faculty of the conscious mind. The conscious mind, in most cases, cannot penetrate the depths to which the subconscious mind has placed the impressions and impulses, and thereby adding logic and reason to these matters buried deep within the memory bank. It is necessary to enter this region by means of the subconscious mind through hypnosis. Once this depth is penetrated, then reason and logic can supplement the disturbing events causing the behavioral responses to be minimized.

Throughout the entire session, including the induction, deepening techniques, and the smoking therapy, the word "sleep" has never been used and did not enter into the conversation. Words that may have a different meaning than that which the hypnotist intends should be avoided until the meaning to be construed is explained, so the subject's understanding corresponds with that of the hypnotist. The word "sleep" in the minds of most persons means being in a restful position with the eyes closed and unaware of the surrounding circumstances or conditions. When a person is in a state of hypnosis, he is not "asleep."

The subject is fully cognizant of all the events taking place within the immediate vicinity. The normal reaction of the subject upon the termination of the session is to remark, "I wasn't hypnotized. I knew everything you said and did, and I heard everything, so I couldn't have been hypnotized," even though this was fully explained to the subject prior to the session.

The hypnotist should be prepared to meet the situation when it comes up, and it will in approximately ninety percent of the cases following the first session. The explanation that the subject will be *aware* at all times during the session *must* precede the hypnotic session and be *confirmed* shortly after the deepening process.

Never use the word "trance."

12

SECOND AND SUBSEQUENT SESSIONS

Each hypnosis session must follow a pre-prescribed plan or pattern. The first and most important principle in hypnotherapy is to utilize only the techniques necessary to produce the result the hypnotist is seeking. If there is no purpose in doing something other than to take up time and make the session longer, forget it.

The first step in any hypnotic session is the *induction*. The end result of induction techniques is eye closure. The subject expects to be hypnotized and so the hypnotist must go through some physical maneuvers to induce the eyelids being closed. Therefore, it is necessary for the hypnotist to develop and master more than one induction technique. The easiest induction technique is to place the hand about 30 inches above the forehead and ask the subject to look into the palm of the hand. As the hypnotist lowers the hand, this invades the space of the subject. And the subject sitting in the chair has no place to go but to close the eyelids. Should the subject's eyes fail to close, just put the hand over the eyelids and the eyelids will close. Use the same induction technique with the subject in subsequent sessions. Varying the induction techniques with the same subject may lead to some confusion.

The second step for *every* session is the *progressive relaxation*. The progressive relaxation is outlined in this book more than once. Master this technique. The progressive relaxation, once mastered, produces results far beyond what most hypnotists may expect. Those practicing hypnosis think that progressive relaxation takes too much time. I demonstrate at seminars that utilizing progressive relaxation, a subject can enter a somnambulism state without any additional deepening techniques. Progressive relaxation is extremely useful when treating addictive symptoms. When it is necessary to utilize additional deepening techniques, progressive relaxation is the only one that is repeated for the same subject. Once any other deepening technique is utilized, the same technique should not be used again on the same subject.

The third step for subsequent sessions (that is, after the first treatment and for special treatment) is to take the subject to the library or any comfort zone, sanctuary, retreat, where the therapy has been given. In normal cases, omit *counting backwards, the classroom, and any other deepening techniques.* Having tested the subject earlier, there is no need for further testing, except when the subject appears to be nervous or exhibit anxiety. All future sessions are carried out in the library or comfort zone. Having done the progressive relaxation properly and having given the subject the posthypnotic suggestions for reinduction, the subject will normally enter into a deeper state of hypnosis with each subsequent session.

Now is the time for the hypnotist to be creative. Use and adapt the library for any one of multiple purposes. In the library, develop a room that has an altar, first aid room, a balcony to toss out unwanted problems, an elevator, or a stairway for additional deepening purposes. Teach self-hypnosis and additional therapy in the library.

For the first hypnotic session, the steps are the following:
- Induction
- Progressive Relaxation
- Counting Backwards from 100 (or another deepening technique)
- Classroom (or another deepening technique)
- Library (removing problems)
- Testing
- New Therapy

For the subsequent sessions the subject is put through the following steps:

- Induction
- Progressive Relaxation
- Library

Having removed the problems and unwrapped the therapy, there is no need to go through the other steps again.

In special cases of treatment such as drug or alcohol addiction, cancer, AIDS, or some other physical disability, the steps may vary. In drug and alcohol treatment, the progressive relaxation is repeated to allow the subject to immediately enter into a deep state of hypnosis. When any session has been terminated *before* all of the steps have been completed, then the next session the subject is returned to the last step before continuing on with the subsequent steps.

For example, should the session proceed with the induction, progressive relaxation, counting backwards from 100, and the classroom, then the next session should be induction, progressive relaxation into the classroom. Now continue from the classroom.

For another example, suppose before the steps have been completed, the session is terminated in the library. Then the next session is as follows: induction, progressive relaxation, and the library. Now continue from the library.

In any event, always go back to the step that was terminated before completion. Every session begins with the induction and progressive relaxation.

Having removed the problems (the books) and unwrapped the new books, these steps do not have to be repeated. Should the subject experience some emotional problems (the same or different problems) between sessions, then the same problem (the same book) may be back on the shelf. These are new experiences, thoughts, or emotions as they relate to the same problem.

As the hypnotist conducts sessions, he will go through a learning experience so that with each session the steps conducted during the sessions are easier and easier. As the hypnotist continues, a strange thing is going to happen to the hypnotist. The hypnotist will be aware that the subconscious mind will talk to him and suggest that certain words should be said or not said, that certain techniques should be used or not used, and when to touch or not touch.

Listen and follow.

13

AGE REGRESSION

One of the basic principles of hypnosis established by modem medical research is that when an individual is exposed to and accepts an idea, impulse, or impression on a subconscious level, his emotional behavior pattern is altered to conform to those matters accepted. So if a person is told his leg is paralyzed and not having rejected the suggestion, he accepts this suggestion in a state of hypnosis. Then he will act accordingly, and this condition will remain until it is removed. Both the suggestion and removal must be during the time when the subject is in a state of hypnosis. This is true whether the suggestions were introduced intentionally or accidentally. A great majority of psychoneuroses and psychosomatic diseases are found in individuals who were accidentally hypnotized and exposed to harmful suggestions while in this state of hypnosis. By utilizing age regression in our therapy, we can remove these harmful suggestions or programs by taking the subject back in time prior to the event that caused the unwanted suggestions to become planted.

Age regression is vital in securing relief from symptomatic difficulties whose origin lies in past events. Once the initial sensitizing event has been established, then logic and reason must be implanted in the memory bank to minimize the importance of this event and to relieve the person from future unwanted automatic responses whose origin was precipitated by this event. The difficulties of the past are tomorrow's burdens, and changes emerge from changes in thoughts.

Hypnosis provides the therapist the means to search within the subconscious mind and reveal accurate recall of early events from the individual's earlier life. During periods of stress, anxiety, shock, high fever, anesthesia, or trauma, the individual loses his normal faculties to analyze the incoming impulses and is helpless to defend himself. An understanding of this mental process that can produce such an irrational response in the human mind, can assist the therapist in solving the problem and preventing such continuous unwanted behavior in the future. To find these troublesome events, the hypnotist must go beyond the history elicited from the patient in his conscious state and go by what is revealed in the hypnotic state. This may require that the individual be age-regressed to an early age in his lifetime, involving a considerable amount of time with the individual to develop his natural ability to enter a very deep state of hypnosis. The nature of the treatment and its duration depend upon the reevaluation of the subject's problems in light of the information brought out during the interrogation while the patient is in the state of hypnosis.

Logic and reason must be added, so the patient can fully understand the basis for his behavior patterns. The patient must be assisted to formulate his conclusions in order that these conclusions may be embedded in the memory bank and with the greatest impact and force, thereby achieving a permanent place in the memory bank. The patient (more than the hypnotist) must participate in the reevaluation process, and a positive mental attitude is essential in order to avoid the possibility of rejection of the suggestion by the patient. Hypnosis does not allow the hypnotist to control the patient's will or mind, but rather it is the means by which the therapist can assist the patient in reinforcing his own will and utilizing the force of the subconscious mind.

Under ordinary circumstances, every normal human being produces emotional reactions on a very reasonable and predictable basis. Upon the happening of an event, a behavioral process commences resulting in an instantaneous emotional pattern. This is true whether the pattern is positive or negative. The whole process evolves around the credibility of the event. When we emotionally experience a recurrence of an event, our emotions are predictable and we may guide our behavior patterns by the beliefs we maintain. Since we direct our emotions by the thoughts and beliefs that we hold, then all that is necessary for change is that we change our thoughts and change our beliefs.

In a hypnotic state, the subconscious mind is sensitized or imprinted through cerebrally transmitted concepts. In an ideal world where the subconscious mind is imprinted with totally positive and supportive "perceptions," the person is at peace with himself. Unfortunately, such is not always the case. For when a person perceives in his mind that a traumatic event is true, even though it may be in fact false, and if his analytical perception is true, then for him it is true. It is this false analytical perception that causes the negative behavioral patterns. The subconscious, not having previously rejected them, accepts the events and perception, and replays these emotions during subsequent events. In many cases, we are unable to cure the problem because we have been unable to find any suitable traumatic event which will explain the origin of the patient's symptoms. Age regression may be the road upon which the hypnotist must lead the patient to search and recall his problems.

There are basically two types of age regression:
1. Memory type
2. Revivification type

The memory type is characterized by poor emotional content with the subject reciting the events like a casual observer. The revivification type is characterized by good emotional content. In the revivification, the event is described in the present tense, exhibiting physiological changes and good results. When the patient uses the *past tense* in expressing his thoughts, he is *remembering* rather than *reliving* those events. Except in very traumatic situations, the patient should be urged to express the events in the present tense and when he stays with it, the emotional content is good and the hypnotist can be reasonably sure that the patient is *living* his past events in his mind.

Whenever the hypnotist determines that age regression is necessary in the treatment, the revivification type (reliving) should be attempted even if it requires additional sessions. Perseverance, repetition, and patience are very important in achieving revivification of a past event; for every small detail of the event should be brought out by constant searching by the hypnotist, especially those details related to sight, sound, and smell. Age regression is nothing more than taking a person back in time.

There are several methods or techniques to create age regression. The hypnotist should master more than one so that when the subject rejects one for any personal reason, there is another one readily available. The better procedure is to take everyone back just prior to the time that the subject experienced the initial sensitizing event. However, in most cases, the time of the event may not be readily available. So I have developed the *library technique* where any person may be regressed to a time in his life when he was a child. Various modifications of the library type may be used by the hypnotist, depending upon the nature of the event to be recalled or uncovered. In addition, included at the end of the chapter are examples of other methods for age regression.

LIBRARY TECHNIQUE

The isle in the library has two sides: (1) a right side, good side, nice side, pleasant side and (2) the other side, not-so-good side, the problem side. Age regression is done on the good side, the nice side, and NOT the other side or problem side. So when the book is opened, there are only nice experiences or good experiences. NEVER, NEVER open up the book on the other side, the not-so-nice side. Opening up a book on the not-so-nice side will reveal pictures of not-so-nice experiences.

The hypnotist should always refer to the right side of the aisle as the good side, nice side, pleasant side, or right side. There is no left side or bad side. The other side is called the "not-so-good-side," "other side," or "problem side."

The books on the shelves on the other side, the not-so-nice side, or the problem side contain ALL of the past experiences as they relate to the title of the book. They contain ALL of the past emotions, feelings and symptoms as they relate to the title of the book. As a therapist, you may also indicate that in the problem book are ALL of the past things they heard, saw, read, or talked about as they relate to the title of the book. Each problem book has a title and these titles could be *Fear, Anxiety, Stress, Smoking, Weight, Drugs, Alcohol*, or any other problem the subject would like to dispose of. It is NOT necessary that the subject relive or experience the past stressful or traumatic experience. On the shelf, it is referred to as a *book*, but as the subject reaches over to the not-so-nice side (the problem side), the subject then takes his *problem* off the shelf. Once the conversion is made from a book to a problem, thereafter always refer to the problem and not the book. (The subject is now holding the *problem*.) The *problem* is then thrown away.

Sometimes it is necessary to regress a person back to an event that is very vague. In such a case, elicit as much information as the person does remember so that there is something that the therapist may start with to build imagery. Assign a title of a book that most describes the event such as auto, jewelry, rape, safe, accident, or any other title with one word. To recall the event, the following steps must be done:

1. Induction
2. Progressive Relaxation
3. Deepening Technique (counting backwards or any other)
4. Second Deepening Technique (classroom or other)
5. Taking the subject to the library (See Chapter 11 on hypnotherapy)

Once the subject is in the library, then continue as follows:

Look around in this library and when you see the bookshelves in rows, nod your head YES that you see the bookshelves in rows.

(The subject nods "yes.")

In a moment, I am going to ask you to select any aisle in this library. Then I am going to ask you to walk over to the aisle and stand between two bookshelves. As you look down the aisle, you find that the books on the right side of this aisle are nice books, good books, and pleasant books. Books on the other side are not-so-nice. So select any aisle, walk over to the aisle, and stand between the bookshelves and look down the aisle. And as you look down the aisle, you find the books on the right side are nice books, good books. Books on the other side are not-so-nice. When you are standing between the bookshelves and looking down the aisle, just nod your head YES that you are standing there.

(The subject nods his head)

As you look down the aisle, all of these books are about you. Everything you did in your entire lifetime is recorded in the books as you look down the aisle. Not only everything you did, but also everything you thought about is also recorded in these books as you look down the aisle. These books also have recorded and do contain everything you have read, what you heard, and what you saw in your entire lifetime. The books on the right side, the nice books, they hold your pleasant experiences, your wonderful thoughts, your good emotions and feelings, symptoms, fantasies, even dreams. So the books on the right side, they hold and contain and have recorded all the nice things you ever did in your whole lifetime ... your beautiful thoughts you had in your whole lifetime, the pleasant feelings and emotions and your nice dreams. The books on the other side, they hold and contain those that ... for you ... haven't been so nice.

The books closest to you, those nearest to you, hold and contain your most recent experiences. That's what you did today, yesterday, and the day before. They have not only your most recent experiences, but also your most recent thoughts. Even your most recent feelings and emotions, your most recent symptoms, fantasies, and dreams are recorded in the books closest to you. The most recent things you saw and what you read and the things you heard are also recorded in the books nearest to you.

The books farther down the aisle are about you when you were younger and smaller. The books farther down the aisle have recorded and do contain the things you did when you were younger and smaller. The thoughts you had when you were younger and smaller are also contained in the books farther down the aisle. Your symptoms, feelings and emotions you had when you were younger are also contained in the books farther down the aisle. The books farther down the aisle also contain the things you heard related to what you saw and read when you were younger and smaller. The books on the far end of this aisle are about you when you were just a baby. So these books on the far end of this aisle contain what you did when you were a baby and what you thought about when you were a baby. All of your feelings and emotions that you experienced when you were a baby are contained in the books at the far end. All of these books that you see down the aisle have pictures, pictures of everything you did in your entire lifetime. And I am not going to ask you what's in any of your books.

Now keeping your eyes on the right side, slowly, very slowly walk down the aisle. Walk about halfway down the aisle and stop. Now reach up on the right side and take a book off the shelf and when you have this book in your hands, nod your head YES that you have this book.

(The subject nods "yes.")

This book is about you when you were younger and smaller. Open this book to a picture when you were younger and smaller. If you need or like, turn the pages and when you see a picture of you doing something nice when you were younger, just nod your head YES.

(The subject nods "yes.")

Still keeping your eyes on the right side, walk all the way down to the end of the bookshelves, stop and then take one small step backwards. Now take a book off the shelf and when you have this book again, nod your head YES that you have this book.

(The subject nods "yes.")

Hold this book in your hands. See, this book is
about you when you were just a baby. So give this book
a hug and a squeeze it to your chest. This book contains
pleasant pictures of you when you were just a baby. This
book is a treasured book of beautiful and wonderful
experiences when you were so very young. Open this
book to a picture of you doing something pleasant when
you were so very young. If you like or care, you may
turn the pages. So when you see a picture of you doing
something pleasant when you were so very young, just
nod your head YES.

(The subject nods "yes.")

Close the book and put the book back on the shelf.

Using this regressive technique, it becomes possible to take
subjects back to the time when they were just babies. Normally
this is a time before their problems started. Should the subject desire
to go back to a prior life, you may continue as follows:

You said that you wish to go back to a prior life. On
the wall, down at the end of the bookshelves is a door.
Now in a moment, I am going to ask you to walk over
to the wall at the end of the bookshelves and when you
see the door again, just nod your head YES that you see
the door.

(The subject nods "yes.")

So go over to the wall at the end of the bookshelves
and stand right next to the door. When you are now
standing next to the door again nod your head, YES, I
AM STANDING NEXT TO THE DOOR.

(The subject nods "yes.")

> Now in a moment, I am going to ask you to open
> the door and when you step through the doorway, you
> step into a pleasant experience that you had in your
> prior life. Open the door and step through the doorway
> and into an experience in your prior life that was for you
> very pleasant. Close the door behind you. Share with me
> where you are and what you see.

Ask, if you like, for details about the subject's prior life experience. Then return the person back to the present by saying:

> I am going to count from one to three and at the
> count of three, you are back in the present time, eyelids
> open, and feeling fine. One ... two ... and three.

Should the subject enter into a traumatic experience and exhibit some abreactions, then quickly state:

> When I clap my hands, you are back in the here and
> now.

Then loudly clap your hands. The subject should instantly open his eyelids and be back in the conscious state. Do not attempt at that time to take the subject back to a prior life. Wait a few weeks and then have the subject go through the same steps; but this time suggest that as he steps through the doorway, he is an observer and only "sees" what is happening and he is not participating in the event. Keep the subject's language in the past tense, for then he is remembering and not reliving the event.

When a person expresses a desire to remember an event that is vague and has very little memory as to the circumstances surrounding the event, then the individual is directed to the "how-and-why" section or the "reference" section of the library.

Regardless what the treatment is to cover, or for what other purpose the individual is to be hypnotized, it is essential that the preliminary steps that lead to the therapy or search be followed.

During the initial, or the first, session there is the induction, progressive relaxation (once or twice), deepening technique (counting backward from 100), a second deepening technique (classroom), and then the library. It is the classroom where imagery is developed. The more work done in the classroom and the more repetitious language that is utilized, the clearer the imagery.

All the prior steps are for the purpose of getting the subject into a deep state of hypnosis to secure success in the therapy conducted in the library. Testing should be done in all cases to insure that the subject is in a state of hypnosis so that the subconscious mind is in the dominant position and the hypnotist's suggestions are, when not rejected, true.

Should an individual express during the interview that he can't remember something or can't find something, then it becomes necessary for the hypnotist to remove and discard the *I-Can't* book as described in the Chapter 11 on hypnotherapy.

A young man came in to see me after being involved in an automobile accident. Following the accident, both cars were driven to a service station and the drivers were to go out to examine the damages. The gentleman that came in to see me entered the service station to report the accident to the police. The other driver got into his car and left. Unfortunately, they never exchanged names or any other information. He was hypnotized and taken to the library, followed the procedure of age regression, and removed the *I-Can't* book. He was taken to the reference section and found the *Auto* book, opened up the book, and saw the license number. Before the day was over, the other driver was arrested for leaving the scene of the accident.

The therapy with reference to this accident was as follows:

Now you know that each of the bookshelves has books on both sides. So go back to the head of the aisle. When you are standing at the head of the aisle again, nod your head YES, so I know that you are at the head of the aisle.

(The subject nods "yes.")

Look at the books on the good side, the pleasant
side, and you know that behind the good books are
another row of books. These books behind the good
books are your reference books. So go over to the next
aisle and look at your reference books. When you are
looking at the reference books, nod your head YES that
you can see your reference books.

(The subject nods "yes.")

I also call this side the how-and-why library, for
these books contain your past experiences that you have
decided to bury so deep, the past events were difficult to
remember. Some of these events could have been buried
so deep by mistake when you were stressed or
frustrated. Now you have decided to access and
remember the past events. So keep your eyes on the
reference side and look around and there is a book that
has the title Auto.

The title of the book represents the circumstances that the
person is now searching. The title could be *Rape, Jewelry, Keys,
Accident, Money, Passport*, etc.

The therapy continued as follows:

When you recognize your Auto book, nod your head
YES that you see your Auto book.

(The subject nods "yes.")

Take your Auto book off the shelf and when you
have this Auto book in your hands, nod your head YES
that you have this Auto book in your hands.

(The subject nods "yes.")

Sit on the floor and put your back to the references books and then put the Auto book on your lap. When you have the Auto book on your lap, nod your head YES. (The subject nods "yes.")

Now in a moment, I am going to ask you to open the cover and when you do, you will find the first page blank. And then I am going to ask you to turn the blank page and on the next page, there is a picture of you in an auto just before the accident. So when you see the picture of you in an auto just before the accident, nod your head YES so I know you see the picture. (The subject nods "yes.")

Open up the cover and the next page is blank. Now turn the blank page and there is on the next page a picture of you in the auto. When you see the picture, just nod your head YES.

(The subject nods "yes.")

I am going to count up to twenty and when I count to twenty, the picture you are looking at comes to life and you see the events that are now taking place. Eighteen ... nineteen ... and twenty.

At the sound of twenty, the therapist should clap his hands loudly. Never start with the number one. The count should be hurried so that the subject doesn't have time to think about anything before the count of twenty is reached. The clapping of the hands makes the subject realize his expectation. As stated in this book, if you want the person to see something definite, you must tell the person what he will see *before* he is in a position to make the observation.

A gentleman came to see me about the combination to his safe. The book he took off the shelf was the *Safe* book. The first page was blank and on the second page was the first number of the combination. The third page held the second number and on the fourth page was the third number.

Should the event be traumatic and stressful, then the subject is told he is an observer and sees the event unfolding before him; and for him, the event is not upsetting, or stressful.

The therapy concluded as follows:

When the event is over, the picture fades away. When the picture is gone, again nod your head, YES so I know that picture is gone.

(The subject nods "yes.")

Close the book and return the book back on the shelf. Now I am going to count up to three and at the count of three, your eyelids do open and you are back in your conscious state, feeling pleasant and fine. One ... two ... and three. Eyes open and feeling comfortable and relaxed.

The library age regression may be adapted in many ways, depending on the need to recall a specific time or period. Keeping the eyes on the right side of the aisle, the subject may randomly select a book and upon examination can picture an event of a previous time. Suggestions of walking farther down the aisle bring the subject to an earlier date. Upon examination of one of the books, the subject recognizes himself at a particular age.

As an example, let's pick age four. Suggestions are then formulated indicating that each book farther down the aisle represents a year earlier and each book back up the aisle is a year later in life. Then having selected the desired year, suggest that each chapter represents a month. Chapter 1 would then be January, and each page in that chapter represents the events of a particular day. Page 2 would be the 2nd of January of the year selected.

The subject is directed to go to the day prior to the day of the event to be revealed. The subject is then instructed that upon turning the page, he does see a picture of the day of the event, beginning in the morning. The picture will come alive so he is seeing the events of the day unfolding before him. He is then instructed to go ahead and turn the page. Upon reciting the events of the day, the subject is directed to use the present tense, reciting as though the events are happening now.

When the event to be recalled has been completed, the book is replaced on the shelf; or if the event is too tragic, the book should be destroyed. It is not necessary to retrace the steps progressively to the present time. Any techniques for returning back to the conscious state may be used to bring the patient to the present time.

ADDITIONAL TECHNIQUES FOR AGE REGRESSION

Auto, Train, or Vehicle Regression: The subject imagines himself entering an automobile, train, or other vehicle, and it is suggested that he is entering into a time machine. As this vehicle proceeds down the road, he finds himself traveling back in time and the scenes he passes along the trail or road are scenes from his earlier days. Suggestions are then given that soon there will appear a curve or a hill in the road and when this point is reached, the subject cannot see the road beyond. *Before* the curve or hill is reached, he is instructed that the desired event is right beyond this point and upon reaching this place, the vehicle does stop and he does get off. Then he describes the details of the event that is taking place. Some subjects may require continuous prodding to bring out details of the event.

Calendar Regression: Suppose something happened on February 10, 1975, that was important and it was necessary to recall the details of the event and that the site of the event was in a building. The subject is then asked to imagine that he is standing in a room of a building similar to the one in which the event took place and in this room is a closed door. Assume, for example, that the event took place in an office building. The subject is then asked to describe the room in which he is standing. Do some prodding or suggesting that there may be items of furniture or equipment such as a desk, chair, pictures, telephone, typewriter, or computer. The more details with which this room can be described, the more details will be in his recollection of the desired event. When the hypnotist is satisfied that the room has been adequately described, then he suggests that behind the subject is a calendar on the wall and this calendar is somewhat different from the regular calendars.

The therapy continues as follows:

> Now in a moment, I am going to ask you to turn around and look at the calendar on the wall. So when you see the calendar on the wall, you do notice that the only thing on this calendar is the current year ...

(You state the current year.)

> Now turn around and when you see the calendar on the wall with the current year on the first page, nod your head YES that you see the page with the current year.

(The subject nods "yes.")

> Now when I clap my hands, the first page falls off and the following pages are the years going backwards to 1976.

(You clap your hands.)

> When you see the number 1976, nod your head YES that you see the number 1976.

(The subject nods "yes.")

Now I am going to clap my hands again and when I clap my hands, the page of 1976 falls off and December appears and December falls off, and the months continue to appear and fall off until March appears and stays.

(You clap your hands.)

When March is on the calendar again, nod your head YES that you see March.

(The subject nods "yes.")

That's fine. Now the next time I clap my hands, March falls off and the number 28 appears and then the number 28 falls off and the pages continue to fall off until the number 10 appears.

(You clap your hands.)

When number 10 remains on the calendar, nod your head YES so I know 10 is on the calendar.

(The subject nods "yes.")

Wonderful. Now it is February 10, 1975, and when you open the door and go through the doorway, you enter a time in February 10, 1975, that you enjoyed. Open the door and enter into an experience that you enjoyed on February 10, 1975. If you like, share with me this experience. When the day is over, it gets very dark. When it is dark, nod your head that it is dark.

(The subject nods "yes.")

I am going to count up to three and when I count three, you are in the here and now. One . ... two ... and three.

Now you may ask questions as to the experiences encountered on that day. Should the desired event that must be recalled have taken place outside any building, as the subject goes through the door of the room with the calendar, he exits to the place where the event happened.

Many individuals are not creative. Therefore, the hypnotist must direct in detail the items comprising the picture and the unfolding events. Explaining in advance the calendar and the falling pages establishes expectations so when the individual turns to look at the calendar, his expectations of the falling pages become a reality and regression is achieved. Anticipation of the events when detailed increases the individual's imagination.

Hypnosis is a change of consciousness. Leave the conscious mind and enter the realm of the subconscious mind to find one's true potential.

14

TREATMENT FOR DRUGS AND ALCOHOL

The human body operates through a delicate but powerful interplay of emotions, produced by the thought created in the conscious and deposited into the brain's memory for future use. Appropriate action is then compelled, based upon this line of thinking, to do whatever is necessary for survival.

Drugs may have what is called "addictive" qualities, but we are not now convinced they are the cause of the intense craving so many users have. So for a moment, let's consider what an "addiction" really is.

Life functions by release of certain powerful chemicals, "drugs" if you will, into the general circulation and neuro-transmitters of the central nervous system. Epinephrine produces anxiety, and the endorphins calm the fears and create relaxation. This delicate anxiety-relaxation balance is the mechanism which keeps us going all day long. It allows us to act, to experience, to create, to feel – in fact, to "live" in the truest sense of the word, and it is as important to us as life itself. A disturbance of this balance is unacceptable.

When an "addictive" drug is ingested, this balance is upset and a state of lethargy results. If, however, the drug is discontinued, the balance gradually returns and the person resumes a more active existence. In order to reestablish this essential balance of the mind-body, two things must be done: (1) increase the output of epinephrine and (2) reduce or shut off the endorphins. If the drug heroin, for example, is withdrawn, the balance swings powerfully in the other direction and the resulting anxiety is so intense, there is a desperate craving for more drugs. Nothing else will do. The person is now "addicted." This, in general, has been the concept underlying addiction and treatment, and considering the dismal performance of this approach, suggested there is more to it than that.

If a drug can, by the means described above, produce a craving for more drugs or as we term it an "addiction," it must work in a reasonable and uniform way on everyone since the human physiology is fairly constant. Yet scientific and our own studies have proved to the contrary. If the urge for drugs is not "addictive," then what is it?

Once you understand how the mind works, the answer to this becomes understandable. It is what is called "compulsion." But since the nature of compulsive behavior is, in general, so poorly understood, it is easier to blame it on something that is understood and is an "addiction." When the nature of compulsive behavior is understood, so is the successful means for dealing with it.

The compulsive act is, to the subconscious mind, a producer or a reminder of survival.

When the threat to survival is perceived by the subconscious, either from a thought created in the conscious or through its own ability to perceive dangerous changes within the body, it "compels" you to do what is necessary to survive. This is done in two ways:

1. It causes an intolerable state of anxiety or fear relative to the urgency of the threat.
2. It creates a conscious picture of the act necessary to relieve the anxiety, which is also the act that leads to survival.

When it gets the message that the act has been completed and survival accomplished, it turns off the anxiety and puts the whole experience in the inactive file.

It is when this final message is incomplete or absent that the subconscious becomes confused. It thinks the original threat is still hanging around somewhere, and it compels the survival act whenever it is reminded of the threat, or compels the survival act at any time, just to be on the safe side.

The understanding of this mind-body relationship is imperative in dealing with alcohol and drug users. It is a medical fact that the brain rules and controls every cell in the human body and that the brain receives only two messages:
1. Excitatory, that is, to do something
2. Inhibitory, that is, to stop doing what it is doing

Everything that happens within the human body is preceded by one of these two thoughts. At the time of birth, the subconscious mind is the dominating force, directing and conveying these messages to the brain. As the child grows and matures, learning to exercise deductive and reasoning powers, the conscious mind takes over the duties, reducing the subconscious mind to the subordinate position.

Survival and dealing with the threat of survival are basically the function assigned to the subconscious mind. Returning the subconscious mind to the position of dominance is the function of the therapist. Once this has been accomplished, the task of treating the user becomes easy. Unfortunately, the present day "experts" in hypnosis aren't familiar with the techniques to accomplish this nor do they know how to conduct tests on the patient to ensure that the patient has achieved this state of hypnosis. Hypnotherapy is useless unless the patient is in a state of deep hypnosis. Whenever the hypnotherapy is unproductive, I blame it on the inefficiency of the therapist.

Our seminars teach the participants the techniques of deep induction, methods of deepening the state of hypnosis, and the therapy necessary for success. The participants learn what to say, when to say it, and how to say it. We leave nothing to chance. We stand by our motto, "We guarantee satisfaction or your money back." In the last nine years, no participant has ever asked for a refund. This success must stand for something. Read the evaluation comments of the participants of the last seminar if there still remains a question.

Drugs and alcohol can provide relief for three basic emotional problems. They are anxiety, depression, and guilt. The problems are not necessarily one or the other but usually a combination of them. We must also recognize that there are really two different and distinct problems that an alcohol or drug user must deal with: one is emotional and the other is physiological. To solve the user's problem, we must go back to its origin.

Why do we have this alcohol or drug problem in the first place? The answer is that we are searching for something we do not now have. This "something" is not physical but emotional. It is the RELIEF or an escape from stress, anxiety, depression, fear, guilt, or some other phobia. Having been a user or an abuser, we have created a physiological problem of imbalance in the body's chemistry. Withdrawal of the drugs or alcohol throws this chemical imbalance in reverse, causing "withdrawal" symptoms. Again there is a search for something we do not now have and the answer is still the same: RELIEF.

This is when it is important to understand the difference between addiction and compulsion. Addiction is the SYMPTOM caused by the chemical imbalance, and compulsion is the RELIEF being sought to remove the symptom.

As an alternative to the general treatment, why not perform surgery to remove these so-called "addictive" symptoms? Since these symptoms are not made of any material and do not occupy any space in the human body, this is impossible. When then is the treatment? This general treatment of removing the alcohol and drugs from the user, together with counseling on a conscious level, has resulted in a dismal record of success. Neither has the success record been any better with the method of weaning, slowly withdrawing the drugs, or substituting a less potent drug. Dealing with the physiological condition and hoping the emotional condition will go away is not the method of treatment.

We have had surgery performed, using hypnosis as the anesthetic, without the patient suffering any pain, anxiety, or stress. As an additional benefit, the healing process required a shorter time period. Periodontal surgery (separating the tissues immediately around the teeth, removing the infected tissues, and possibly performing jaw bone reconstruction) is a painful, stressful, and emotional experience if performed without an anesthetic. This surgery was done without the benefit of any chemical anesthetic, using hypnosis only. It doesn't make any difference if this physical change is a result of any chemicals or a surgeon's knife. Treat the emotional problem and let the body's chemistry take care of the physical problem.

An important issue to deal with is a better understanding of hypnosis, especially how it works. What we truly believe is what is going to happen and since most of the users are at the end of the line for so many that have failed before, belief can be a little shaky.

At the initial interview, a detailed history is taken, especially focusing on the previous attempts and treatments to remove this compulsion. This is followed by a lengthy explanation of how and why hypnosis works. When the user understands our concept of hypnosis, he is given the option whether or not to continue with the treatment.

The next thing that must be done is to explain the success rate of this type of treatment. This must be done scientifically and confidentially. Since most of our patients have been referred, at least for us, this has not been a difficult task. The user must be given a plausible reason why he has failed previously and why he is now going to succeed. In the past, most of the patients have been told and accepted that their failure was due to the fact that they were hopeless addicts. Now they begin to understand their own experience as to the nature of compulsions and that compulsions can be broken.

When the user elects to continue the program, he must attend sessions on several consecutive days. There are two sessions on the first and second day, and these sessions may last up to three hours each. These sessions are normally devoted to inductions and deepening techniques. Depending upon the responses of the user, therapy may be instituted on the second day. The first session of the third day is devoted almost entirely to therapy. The second session of the third day, the patient is taught self-hypnosis. On the fourth and fifth days, the patient performs self-hypnosis in the presence of the instructor who supervises and continues to add additional therapies as the sessions progress. The sessions for the third, fourth, and fifth days last from two to three hours. After the fifth day, the sessions (if required) may vary, depending on the patient's motivation, ability, desire, and responses to suggestion.

Our experience has shown that upon completion of the first day's sessions, the "compulsive" behavioral symptoms should be minimal and following the second day's sessions, the "compulsive" behavior or "addictive symptoms" should be almost eliminated. At this time, the patient feels so good, he may think he is "cured" and consequently fail to attend any further sessions. This is why we require payment in full in advance to eliminate this false sense of security and non-completion of the entire program. As long as the user has paid for the sessions, he will attend the sessions scheduled. All of the patients are advised in advance that should they terminate the program, there are no refunds and should the program be interrupted, they must start from the beginning and pay an entire new fee. This has eliminated late cancellations and no-shows.

Some of our successful patients include a federal judge, a circuit judge, two U.S. senators, four local officials, three movie stuntmen, three professional basketball players, four professional football players, five psychologists, two physicians, and six university professors.

Initially, some insurance companies have considered our program as experimental and have objected to payment but as this program has developed and our success rate increased, their position has changed. We now have a backlog of cases upon which we can rely.

Contrary to general opinion, hypnosis (whether it is applied in the field of medicine, forensic or investigative, clinical or therapeutic) is not a complicated or complex endeavor. We have always maintained and do express that once understood, hypnosis is the easiest and safest method of treatment. Most of the persons involved in the health field are there because they have a genuine desire to participate in the treatment of those suffering, and most of them understand their limits. Every day we receive calls from throughout the country from physicians, psychologists, and hypnotherapists inquiring as to the method of treatment of given conditions. Even the professionals know their limitations.

One of our patients had a difficult time removing stress following an automobile accident. On two occasions he attempted suicide. When he was regressed back to the time of the accident, he remarked that the paramedic has stated to an assistant, "This guy is as good as dead so let's look after the other person." When we dealt with this remark during the hypnotic session, his recovery was complete. A remark by a surgeon during the course of surgery, "This boy will never walk again," left the patient paralyzed for over two years.

So where do we draw the line in our teachings?

Hypnotherapy treatment of users of drugs and alcohol follow a parallel pattern. The successful hypnotic sessions depend upon a thorough, full, and complete interview. The interview must include information as to the length or time the person has been using the drugs or alcohol, how often per week or per day, where the substance has been used, and with whom. You may ask from whom the substance is obtained, but don't be surprised when you don't get a truthful answer. The hypnotist must take copious notes, for these notes will be used to formulate the nature of treatment.

The old but still persistent theory is to first get the chemicals out of the body and then treat the emotional problem. Considering the miserable success, one wonders why some therapists insist this is the only method of treatment: Confine the individual to a rehab center for thirty days and allow the body to purge itself of the chemicals and then counsel the patient as to the benefits of not using the drugs or alcohol. I have had patients who come in to see me and had as much as sixty days in a rehabilitation center only to search for the drugs or alcohol the day of the discharge.

During the last fifteen years at my seminars, I have been told by the participants that it is the body that demands the chemicals. Without the drug or alcohol, the addictive symptoms cannot be alleviated. Most patients will rob, steal, and fight to secure the drug or alcohol. In their minds, the called "addictive" symptoms such as sweating, aching, anxiety, pain, fear, etc., can only be removed when the alcohol and drug has been consumed. Take the drug and remove the craving and give the person his relief. What a loss of time and efforts.

There is one of two basic reasons for a person to be on drugs or alcohol:

1. The individual has been involved in a traumatic incident sometime in his life, probably at an early age
2. The person's self-esteem is at a very low level

In the first interview, the therapist/ hypnotist must search for the answer. Don't be surprised if the answer is not at that time uncovered. Ask as many questions as to how, when, why, where, with whom or any other question that might shed some light on the use of drugs or alcohol. Should the subject at any time feel uneasy or threatened by any question, then just back off. As we go along in this chapter, I will show you how to obtain the answers without any difficulty.

The hypnotist has only one goal in mind: to treat the urge and compulsion, to take the drug and alcohol, and to give the person some relief from the symptoms that are now being manifested in the body.

The duration of the time the person has been using the drug or alcohol and the amount used, have a decided effect upon the symptoms experienced. The longer the usage and the more consumed, the greater the symptoms. What are the thoughts that the individual entertains? "I need a 'fix' or a drink and that will take care of my symptoms." This is the message the brain must process into the body.

By now you should have realized what we're getting into. Change the thought and change the symptom.

A patient of mine underwent a two-hour periodontal surgery without the use of any chemical anesthetic. The patient was in the

274 Medicine of the Mind

dentist's chair while the dentist surgically removed the gums from the jaw bone. The dentist then proceeded to remove the bone spurs, cleanse the teeth, extracted one tooth, and cut out the infected tissues. Sixty-four stitches were required to replace the gums back to the jaw bone. Anesthesia was created by suggestive hypnotic therapy. The numbness remained until the healing was complete. The bleeding was minimal. What was removed was a symptom called pain. I have treated hundreds of patients for pain while the body was in a damaged condition. Childbirth can be painful yet with the proper suggestions, it can be painless and occur with ease and comfort.

What the hypnotist treats is the symptoms and not the body. Understand there are no cells in the body that are pain, fear, anxiety, depression, love, joy, or urge and compulsion. The symptoms are a product of the thought process. Change the thought and change the symptom.

During the initial visit, the subject should be given a thorough explanation of what hypnosis is all about. In addition, the number of visits are outlined and explained in detail. The amount of your fee is to be laid out in advance and there are no guarantees that your services will be successful. Follow the steps in this book and success will be accomplished. Get your full payment in advance before you set the first session. Take it from me: if you agree to take payments in installments, the first payment will usually be the only one you get. Set the schedule and remind the subject that any no-shows will be charged extra.

Most of the users of drugs and alcohol are already in a light state of hypnosis due to their stressful lifestyle. A simple induction of eye closure is sufficient. However, before the hypnotist undertakes a session, a plan of treatment must be laid out for each subject. Everyone responds differently. This plan of treatment is constructed after the initial visit.

Your primary schedule should be conducted with two sessions for the first two days, and thereafter should be conducted in a single session on the days you meet.

DAY ONE, SESSION ONE

- Induction
- Progressive Relaxation
- Second Progressive Relaxation
- Third Progressive Relaxation

These Progressive Relaxations should be done from the eyelids down to the toes. No exceptions.

- Deepening Technique (counting backwards from 100)
- Returning the subject back to the conscious state by counting from one to three

Send the subject out for lunch or coffee and have the person return in about one and a half hours.

DAY ONE, SESSION TWO

- Induction
- Progressive Relaxation
- Second Progressive Relaxation
- Deepening Technique (classroom)
- Following the deepening technique (A, B, C, D, etc.), send the subject to a chair in the classroom and conduct a second interview, just like the first one but in more detail.

You may get the information that eluded you in the first interview. The subject's language and expressions will be different from the first interview. Take and keep extensive notes. This information can be used during the therapy session.

- Return the subject back to conscious state by counting from one to three.

Send the subject home and have him return the next day. In one day, the subject has gone through four or five progressive relaxations so by this time, he should be extremely relaxed. The past addictive symptoms should not be as severe.

DAY TWO, SESSION ONE

- Induction
- Progressive Relaxation
- Second Progressive Relaxation
- Take the subject to the classroom.
- Then take the subject to the library.
- Age regress the subject on the right side, good side, nice side, all the way down to a baby or small child.
- Take the subject to the other side, not-so-good side.
- Remove the books *Stress*, *Fear*, *Pain*, *Alcohol*, *Drugs*, *I-Can't*, *Excuses*, and any other book (problem) that may be elicited during the second interview.
- Send the container and problems out of the library.
- Take the subject to a chair in the library and explain what has been done. (See Chapter 11 on hypnotherapy.)
- Test the subject for depth of hypnosis.
- End the session by counting up to three.

Send the subject out for lunch or coffee and have the person return in about one and a half hours.

DAY TWO, SESSION TWO

- Induction
- Progressive Relaxation
- Take the subject to the library.
- Send the subject to the good side, right side, and unwrap the books entitled *Health* and *Happiness*, *Success*, and *Desires*.

Since every problem has its own book, so too every need or benefit can have its own book. Create titles depending upon the needs developed during the second interview.

- Return the subject back to the chair in the library.
- Now is the time to do the testing for depth.
- Follow the testing techniques explained in Chapter 11 on hypnotherapy or Chapter 9 on testing.
- Conduct the therapy.

The following therapy deals with drugs. When you are working with a subject who has a particular drug problem, name that drug each time you refer to the drug. Substitute the word "alcohol" in place of "drug" when working with an alcoholic.

Proceed as follows:

Now, you do some serious thinking. And if you want to be a particular kind of person, you have to tell yourself, " I am." So as you are in a nice, comfortable position, you just think to yourself, "I never used to be, but I am now the most relaxed person in the whole world." When you make this statement, you may not be relaxed because the response comes after you send the message. And the more often you send the message, the faster you become that kind of person. So what you are going to do is to keep compounding these messages.

You are saying, "Brain, guess who I am, not who I used to be. And listen to me, I am the most relaxed person in the whole world. You bet I am. And let me explain how nothing bothers me anymore. Nothing. Nobody. Nobody upsets me. Nobody steals my time, nobody steals my energy, nobody steals my efforts. They're mine, I keep them. And I am the one in charge of everything I do in my whole lifetime, just me. I'm responsible for what I do. I'm in charge of what I do, and I'm in charge of what I think about. I control my emotions, my symptoms, my feelings. Nobody else, just me. Nothing, nobody, just me."

So you think, "I am the most relaxed person anybody could meet." Besides being so relaxed and so comfortable, if you want to be, you just tell yourself, "I'm a compassionate person. I'm a caring person." If you want to be, you tell yourself, "I'm a joyful and happy person. When I look around, I find all goodness around me. I'm only interested in the good things in this life." And if you want to be, you tell yourself, "I am confident, I'm capable, capable beyond most person's expectations. That's me." And if you want to be, you tell yourself, "I'm successful in everything I do." If you think you are, I've got news for you: that's who you become.

It all begins with your thought. You see, your problem is you've been criticizing yourself saying, "What the hell's wrong with me? Why can't I do something right? Why do I have to get myself involved in all these things? I guess my willpower is shot. I'm a failure anyway." And that's all the brain could process and program for you. And guess what? You became the sum total of your thoughts.

And so if you want to be somebody different, you have got to tell yourself, "I'm somebody different. But

let me tell you who I am. Successful? Oh, you bet I am."
It may be a false statement when you make it, but the
truth comes after the message because now the brain
has something to work with. You have to give the brain
food for thought, to work with, process and program.
So understand, you can be any kind of person you want
to be. Any kind. But it begins when you send the brain a
message, "I am." Then you explain in detail specifically
the kind of person you are. And you don't have to do
anything you don't want to do.

God gave you the right to make a decision. To do or
not to do. He gave you a right to exercise your
discretion, that is, to make choices. Just you. But a lot
of people, you know what they do? They create excuses,
just a lousy, rotten excuse to justify their conduct. You
see, you never used any drugs until you first thought
about it. Oh yes, then you went and got it. Then you
put it in your body. You did that. It can make you feel
better, but it didn't. For a moment probably. Later on,
things got worse and worse and you needed more drugs
and more drugs and things got worse and worse and
more drugs. And you were on a slide. Big slide, slide
that was greased. And you decided to get off this slide.

And I say to you, "To change your conduct, you
have to first change how you think." You have to send
new messages to the brain so the brain can do
something new to your body.

And so you sit in that comfortable place where you are and you tell yourself, "Me, I never do drugs anymore. Oh no, I'm a non-user. I have no desire. I have no need for drugs. Not today, not tomorrow, not ever." Any kind of drugs. Amphetamines, cocaine, heroin. What difference? They're all drugs. All destructive and it's not for you. You see, your body is too precious. Your body is the most important thing you are ever going to own in your whole lifetime. Time you started taking care of that body of yours.

You see, when you take care of yourself, then you can help others. You can be a member of your family. Productive, caring, compassionate, constructive. I told you it begins with you and how you think. And you tell yourself, "No, no. The very thought of me using drugs, the very thought of it causes my whole body, every cell in my body to literally scream at me. Get it out of here. Doesn't belong in here. Don't want it."

And all you have to do is send a whole new message. All you have to do is say, "Me, I don't do drugs anymore. I have no desire for drugs. My body is too precious to put drugs in there. Each and every thought rejecting the use of drugs causes me to feel comfortable, content, and thoroughly satisfied in my whole mind and my whole body." Each subsequent time, that means every time, you reject the use of drugs causes you to feel progressively more pleasant, more comfortable, more peaceful, more successful, and more confident in your whole body from the top of your head, all the way down to your toes. Every thought rejecting the use of drugs and every word you use rejecting the use of drugs causes every cell in your whole body to slowly and progressively relax and settle down. Recognize and realize that you have finally taken control and complete charge of yourself. When you are driving around or just walking, you think, "I have finally taken control of myself and I sure love who I am."

So when you think about the times when you used to use the drugs and the persons who were present, you just tell yourself, "These people are off limits for me. I cannot get along with people who push me to the brink of death. They used to be good friends but friends don't kill one another."

And when you think about the supplier of drugs and the places you visited for drugs, this causes your stomach muscles to tighten and it squeezes the stomach muscles like a ball being squeezed. This tightening of the stomach muscles causes the bile in your stomach to come up your esophagus and up into your throat. The sensation of the squeezing and taste of the bile cause your whole body to become nauseated and uncomfortable. The supplier of drugs is out to kill you and not to comfort you. Each and every time you see or think about your supplier, this causes you to feel progressively more nauseated and upset. And so, too, each and every time you reject seeing your supplier, this causes you to feel more comfortable, satisfied, and content.

Understand that you are protecting your precious body, the most important thing you are ever going to have. The places where you used to buy the drugs are off limits, and you feel comfortable and content not going there. The persons you used to associate with doing drugs are off limits. No matter how close they used to be, they are always off limits. That means you don't associate or meet with them. Not today, tomorrow, or ever.

Hey, life is pleasant. It really is. Life is rewarding. You see, you have finally decided you are important, more important than the friends who were involved in drugs. You are the most important person in the whole world. And that's the person you take care of from today and every day. When you take care of yourself and you are strong, then you can help others.

Life is what you make it by how you think. It is always back to the basic thing. It is your mind, your brain, and your body. It is yours, it belongs to you. You control your body in whatever you do. Survival is the most important thing in your whole lifetime. To live. To create. To do. To enjoy.

- Finally, return the subject back to the conscious state by counting from one to three.

Send the subject home and have him return the next day for one session.

DAY THREE AND AFTER

- Induction
- Progressive Relaxation
- Take the subject to the library. (Every session hereafter, always take the subject to the library.)
- Teach self-hypnosis. (Follow the instructions on self-hypnosis as outlined in Chapter 16.)

The subject should come in every third or fourth day after learning self-hypnosis so you can monitor how well the subject is progressing. After two weeks, the subject should come in once a week for two months. Thereafter, taper off the sessions. Each individual will proceed differently so the sessions, after learning self-hypnosis, can vary.

Twenty hours is a fair average for the treatment for drugs and alcohol. Multiply the hours by the fee per hour you find necessary to carry on your business and you get an estimate of the total charges for your treatment.

15

SPECIAL TREATMENT

The hypnotherapeutic treatment of any symptomatic condition follows a precise pattern. Hypnosis is not a cure, but the means by which a cure is developed. This treatment, whether it be for a change in physical responses or emotional symptoms, should follow a prescribed pattern of five precise steps:

- Relaxation
- Recognition
- Removal
- Reeducation
- Reinforcement

Each of these steps must be carried out by the hypnotist in this order to provide adequate and competent treatment of the patient.

Prior to the initial session, the hypnotist must acquaint himself with the nature of the difficulty of the patient and work out a plan of treatment and nature of the suggestions to be given. Changes or modifications may be in order after the personal interview only when some of the new and dramatic events are brought to light. Most new information will be cumulative with events in which the responses or emotions reoccur; the times and places change but not the symptoms. This information can be dealt with at subsequent times.

The patient must enter into a state of relaxation before any attempt is made to use hypnotherapy as a means of treatment. The more severe the symptom or condition, the deeper the state of hypnosis. Recognize that any induction technique is only the entrance step into hypnosis. When the hypnotist has reason to believe the patient has achieved the depth necessary for the nature of treatment, testing may begin. Any time the test produces a negative response, additional deepening techniques must be employed until the proper depth is recognized. In most cases when the induction is followed by progressive relaxation and one deepening technique, that state of relaxation is adequate; at each subsequent session, a deeper state will automatically happen.

One must recognize, however, that the patient's depth may vary during the course of the session without the hypnotist being fully aware of this variation. To guard against this, use simple cumulative suggestions for relaxation intermittently, such as that the passing of time, each moment causes the patient to relax progressively more and more or that the sound of a voice, clock, or motor causes the patient to go deeper and deeper into relaxation.

Prior to the initial session, the patient must have a conscious commitment and a desire for a change from the undesirable conduct or symptom. It then becomes the hypnotist's duty to direct the patient so the cause of this difficulty is revealed. This recognition may be developed regressively or progressively – that is, working backwards beginning with the most recent event and going back to the very first occurrence, or beginning with the first time the patient remembers his participation in the symptom and working forward to the most recent occurrence.

One of my stressful patients had a need to lose ninety pounds and even though we were able to reduce her food consumption by one-half, she didn't lose a proportionate amount of weight. Subsequent sessions revealed that fifteen years earlier, her first husband was institutionalized with a severe depressive attitude, leaving her to raise a baby and support the family alone. Even though each visit to the hospital was depressing, she made three visits each week. On the way home from each visit, she stopped at a delicatessen and bought some cheesecake. After putting the child to bed, she sat at the kitchen table and slowly ate the cake, savoring each bite. This food was her reward for living through this stressful situation. Her family situation, at the time of her treatment, was no different. She worked in a business with her second husband which she considered intolerable, and her two teenage daughters made her life so miserable, she was planning on moving out of her home. During these sessions, she came to recognize and realize that her present eating pattern was a repetition of the earlier one, one related to stress. Recognizing that all prior attempts to change both the business relationship as well as the relationship with her daughters were fruitless, she learned to accept them as unchangeable situations. Since she couldn't do anything about these stressful situations, she might just as well be thin; for in that condition, she could reward herself by buying new clothes and improving her appearance in fulfillment of her desires. Within ten days, she lost sixteen pounds, and the pounds continued to "melt off."

Reoccurrence of the symptoms is directly related to the importance of the initial event. The greater the importance assigned to the event, the more frequently the symptom will recur. In addition, there is a greater probability that the number of associated events will increase. For example, should the event of sexual molestation be very traumatic, then in all likelihood subsequent contact in later years with a similarity of room, furniture, curtains, paintings, or rugs can easily cause the subject to experience symptoms similar to those experienced at the original event.

During the session, the patient is asked to illicit what triggered the disturbing symptoms. Several associated causes may be responsible, so each must be dealt with separately. At each such revelation, the importance must be minimized by using logic and reason. Reducing the importance not only reduces the recurrences, but also the severity of the symptoms. Simple, framed suggestions are usually more effective than long, drawn-out sentences or the use of unfamiliar technical or medical terms. Such suggestions may be stated as follows:

With each passing year, our values change in the
light of our new circumstances and surroundings. Some
things that were important then are no longer
important. When you were very young, you played with
dolls or jacks (boys – with marbles or baseballs) and
at that time, you found these things to be the most
important things in your life. But as you grew older,
these things fell by the wayside and you found other,
more important things to do. These events that we
talked about that caused you those disturbing symptoms
were a long time ago. So why don't you just think that it
may have been important to you then, but that passing
of time has changed how you now appraise the situation
and you do not find it very important but a thing of the
past? Since it is of the past, why not just drop it so it
doesn't clutter up tomorrow's pleasures?

Reeducation or reevaluation is primarily directed to the
person's perception of a sensitizing event at the time of its inception.
Once this perception has been recorded in the memory bank of the
subject, it and its corresponding symptoms or emotions emerge
with every recollection of the event of the associated events.
Subsequently, we find the subject continuously on a conscious level
seeking a solution for these undesirable responses and when a
solution is not readily available, one suffering from stress or anxiety
may seek refuge in alcohol or other drugs. Children may resort to
enuresis to gain attention or affection, while others may suffer
psychosomatic pain to obtain sympathy or reward. Unfortunately,
once established and maintained, these problems are not easily
removed, hence the sessions with the hypnotist.

Reeducation consists of evaluating the causes of these
disturbing symptoms and the unwanted conduct in the light of

present-day circumstances; for as things change, so do our values. Treatment utilizing reeducation produces better results when working in the reverse order, taking a look at the desired results first. A decision must be made as to the future goals of the subject, then what changes must be made to accomplish these goals. Stress and anxiety are not causes but results of a perception by the individual that a situation is uncontrollable and that there is nothing that can be done about it. Treatment then consists of medication, alcohol, or other drugs in an attempt to relieve this stress. This treatment is only temporary, for the cause of the condition always remains.

The road to success in any hypnotherapeutic treatment means keeping paramount in the subject's mind the ultimate goal to be achieved, for the subject must have already developed a belief that in his mind the goals have already been achieved and it is merely time for the body to follow his psychological picture. Most problems have their origin in unintentional or accidental hypnosis – that is, when the subconscious mind, not having rejected them, accepts impressions, events, and perceptions without the benefit of logic or reason. Hypnotizing the person sends him back to that state of hypnosis that allowed this to happen. Then adding logic and reason to the unfolding events gives rise to new and different impressions and perceptions, relieving the person of the difficulties.

Although the factual situations are the same, our responses and attitudes differ due to the new perceptions. Attack the initial cause with a double-barreled approach of reason and logic. Everything can be logical under new and different circumstances, and since time has already passed since the initial event, things have changed. No situation need be stressful unless it is perceived and accepted as such. What may have been before need not be now.

When we search and ask for a solution, one is available to every problem. However, when a person accepts the idea that the problem is unsolvable, stress, failure, and physical deterioration soon follow. The flight syndrome must be reversed by reeducation of the person to accept the challenge of each and every problem.

Search for a solution by using simple logic and reason, anticipating the feeling of success. Worry solves no problems. Lead the way with positive and corrective suggestions, restoring the patient's confidence and self-image.

These positive suggestions must be continuously reinforced through the use of self-hypnosis. Reinforcement by means of repetition develops success. The person should always be encouraged to carry out his commitment for change. Self-hypnosis should be an integral and vital element of treatment. No person should be denied these benefits.

The mind doesn't really care what or how much it stores, nor does it care if the events unfolding are real or imagined; for once stored while in the state of hypnosis, these events for that individual are real. Whether real or imagined, if repeated often enough during the self-hypnotic sessions, they are then stored as real memories.

I have developed a formula for the treatment of ALL emotional and symptomatic problems. Symptomatic problems do not exist in the body in any form, shape, or manner. There is no cell, gland, or tissue that is depression, fear, anger, hate, love, joy, anxiety, happiness, or any phobia. These are all products of our thinking process. How we perceive a situation causes our body to respond. If we perceive danger, then our body experiences stress and uncertainty. Should we perceive a situation as pleasant and comfortable, then we experience a feeling of relaxation and joy.

Since we respond to perceptions, then changing the perception changes the responses. How we think is so important. Since all the things we do (our events) are preceded by a thought, and all of our emotions, symptoms, and feelings are preceded by a thought, then all we need to do is change how we think. When we change how we think, then we change what we do and how we feel.

So what does it take? Only a thought.

While in a state of hypnosis, intentionally or unintentionally, unless the statement, perception or thought is rejected, it is accepted and deposited in the brain as *absolutely true*. The deeper the state of hypnosis, the greater the certainty of the response.

Removing the problems by disposing of the books in the library (or using any other method) does not in itself create new and different responses. It then becomes the responsibility or duty of the therapist to create a change in the responses to the thought or circumstances.

The formula for treatment is as follows:

The subject must think about something or do something that causes the intended result, or the therapist must do something or say something that causes the intended result. The first thing to be determined is the result that is desired. The *something* used in the formula or treatment need not be related to the result. The suggestion may be any of the following:

(1)

As you think about moving your leg, your thoughts cause your leg to grow numb and useless.

(2)

As you think about the pain in your back, your thoughts cause the pain in your back to fade away and disappear.

(3)

As you think about going into an elevator, your thoughts cause you to feel totally relaxed and at ease.

(4)

As you enter into the elevator, each step you take causes you to feel relaxed, comfortable, and safe.

(5)

As you listen to the music, each note causes you to feel comfortable and more and more relaxed.

(6)

Each step you take to stand before the class to give your talk causes you to feel more and more comfortable.

(7)

Each word you speak before the group causes you to feel more comfortable and at ease.

(8)

Each passing moment causes you to feel better and better, more relaxed and secure.

(9)

As I gently stroke your arm at the elbow, this causes the pain in your elbow to fade away and disappear.

(10)

As I gently touch your forehead, this causes the pain in your head to disappear.

This formula is used quite often when testing for depth of the person being treated.

PAIN

In medical practice the need to relieve apprehension and anxiety has always been recognized. In the treatment of pain, hypnosis has been found to be quite reliable in replacing drugs without the danger of addiction. Pain is only the interpretation of the sensations of pressure, touch, temperature, and disturbance. This interpretation is our perception based upon past experiences, knowledge, and environment. When we perceive a situation to be painful, we tend to realize our expectation and, therefore, enhance our painful experiences. Recognize, then, that our perceptions are valuable in changing pain sensations.

Pain is merely a message from one part of the body alerting the brain that something is wrong. It makes no difference to the person whether the message of pain is psychological or physiological. In either case, the person suffers this debilitating symptom. No attempt should be made to remove any pain symptom until the cause has been determined. Once this cause has been ascertained, treatment may begin. The removal procedure is the same for real pain as for psychosomatic pain, as the human body suffers equally from both. The patient is unable to determine the difference, for the symptom to him is real in either case.

Psychosomatic pain is the result of how we think and what we think about. In every case, the key for removing pain is complete relaxation, followed by therapeutic suggestions. (The threshold of pain is raised in proportion to the relaxation created.) Both hypnosis and narcotics deliver the same response; both enable the person to ignore the pain.

It is important to dwell on the amount of success, even if minimal, when conversing with the patient, pointing out to him that he has achieved the ability to ease the pain. All that remains is for him to develop the power within to control all levels of his own pain.

Nowhere does the right choice of words mean so much as in hypnosis. Words with more than one meaning or possible interpretation should be avoided. Especially in the treatment of pain, the subject must be reminded that he must remain alert and aware, and that he must listen, hear, and remember each of the instructions given by the hypnotist.

In many cases of psychological pain, there is an underlying conflict that is suppressed. Medication only temporarily relieves the symptom which will flare up again and again. Psychological pain is relatively simple to correct. All that is usually required is to create anesthesia in the hand or leg, then transfer this feeling to the area or pain together with suggestions for removal of the symptom. Apply water or lotion to the area affected with the suggestion that this material is something very special and its application causes the pain to terminate. Even suggestions of complete cure can be implemented. Should this type of treatment be used, then under no circumstances should the patient be informed of the true nature of the material applied. In most cases where the patient learns of the true nature of the material, the pain automatically returns and sometimes is more severe. To some persons, this may appear unethical; however, one must understand that one must take extreme measures to remove the suffering, which in most cases is extremely debilitating.

The procedure for the removal of pain, psychosomatic or physiological, is somewhat the same. In either case, the patient is age-regressed to locate the initial sensitizing event and all associated events. Physiological pain can be caused either by stress or trauma and in every case, there is some damage to the organic structure of the human body; for stress is a component in every disease. In age regression, I personally prefer to use the library method, for this allows the patient to search and very easily find his cause or causes. These causes are then removed and discarded.

Every problem has its own book. Using any one of the induction techniques and deepening processes, the patient imagines he is in a library, looking down between the bookshelves. On the right side of this aisle are the good books representing those events in his life that are pleasant, and on the other side are books representing those events that are not so good. He is then asked to walk down the aisle, picking up and looking into the books that represent his past, until he has reached a period of time in his life that precedes the commencement of the problem. When this period has been reached, he is then asked to look at the books on the other side, which are problem books, to search for the book that represents his present problem.

These suggestions may be stated at follows:

Look on the not-so-good side, and there is a book called Pain. Find that book. It is there. That book holds all of the events that caused the pain you now experience and all of your thoughts about this disturbing and discomforting symptom. Since it is not tied down to any cell or organ, why don't you just get rid of it? Find that book, and when you find it, take the Pain book off the shelf and just nod your head that you have it.

(The subject nods his head.)

Look around on the floor of this aisle, and you will find a container. When you see this container, take the Pain book over to it and throw it in that container. When you have thrown the Pain book away in that container, again nod your head so that I know you have thrown it away.

(The subject nods his head.)

This is then followed with directions to find the *I-Can't* and *Excuses* books, together with any other problem books. All these books are removed from the library and destroyed as previously outlined. Then the patient is directed to sit in the library chair and reflect upon what has been accomplished. Since pain is only a symptom and is not made of any material, does not occupy any space, and cannot be touched, recognize that it is like a spirit. It is made by the subconscious mind in its own image.

Since the subconscious mind created this pain, it can now take it away; for it is only a message. It is now time to disconnect this message of what now is harmless pain, for this continued message now serves no useful purpose.

In a few moments, I am going to ask you to look around in your library and you will find an electrical box on the wall. You know what an electrical box is. It's one that holds all of the fuses and breaker switches, just like in your house. These switches are like an ordinary light switch. All of these switches in this box have markings on them, indicating the direction of the flow of energy. These switches may be labeled back, arm, leg, head, or any other part of your body.

Now look around in your library and find that electrical box and when you see it, just nod your head. (The subject nods his head.)

Go over to that box, open the cover, and find the switch that is labeled back (or any other area that is being treated). Put your fingers on the switch, but don't move it. When you are touching the switch, again nod your head.

(The subject nods his head.)

The switch in this position allows the message of harmless pain to be sent from your troubled area. Just like a light switch that allows energy to flow to the light bulb, when this switch is moved in the other position, the energy stops and the light goes off. By flipping this switch in the other position, you cut off the human energy and the message of harmless pain.

Now when I clap my hands, you flip the switch. (The therapist claps his hands.)

Let yourself relax. Really let go and relax. Think of relaxation and as you do so, these thoughts cause the troubled area to become progressively more and more relaxed, more numb, and feeling better and better. Release the pain and let it go. Shut down the message and relax.

Another very simple and useful technique is to substitute a telephone for the electrical box. Upon seeing the telephone, the patient will notice that the phone is off the hook or cradle. All that remains to be done is to replace the phone so the message of pain is disconnected. Remember to describe all circumstances and conditions before the patient is instructed to imagine anything and before the suggestions to perform are given.

INSOMNIA

Insomnia, like all other symptoms, has its own initial sensitizing event. However, here we can easily discover these events; for they usually are recognized by the patient. Fear and worry are the predominate causes of insomnia. Some patients may be reluctant to reveal the cause or causes during the pre-induction talk. However, when the patient is in a state of hypnosis, suggest that he share with you, the hypnotist, these causes so that together they can be discovered. Sharing seems to ease the patient's apprehension about revealing his deep-seated emotions and events. Fear of dying in sleep or fear of facing tomorrow's events represents the majority of reasons for insomnia.

As in most therapies, the hypnotist should insert positive suggestions, minimizing the importance of these fearful events to break up the habit pattern. Leave no room for doubt that this pattern can be interrupted and destroyed. In some respect, pain and insomnia are related; for as long as the patient suffers pain, he is still alive and as long as the person is aware, there is life. Patients usually assess their problems in light of their own experiences.

A feeling of uselessness or unimportance in older persons brings about restless nights and little sleep. Suggestions establishing importance and creating meaningful activities make life more pleasant and reduce the recurrence of sleepless nights.

Make a simple suggestion, such as having the patient make a list of all of his friends, then inquire as to their desires. At night, the patient should then pray that these friends achieve their desires. As the number of friends grows, the more mentally active the client becomes so that there isn't time or energy to be concerned about loneliness.

Falling asleep is a function assigned solely to the subconscious mind, for one cannot consciously fall asleep. By actively trying to fall asleep, the function of the subconscious mind is interrupted.

Suggest while the patient is in a state of hypnosis that falling asleep requires no effort or energy; therefore, it is easy to allow the subconscious mind to create a condition of relaxation and sleep. Follow this with suggestions that each and every time the patient rests his head on the pillow, this is a suggestion of relaxation and that upon such an event the subconscious mind is instructed to relax the body and allow the person to enter into a state of natural sleep.

To use the formula for insomnia, the suggestion may be as follows:

As you think about going to bed to sleep for the evening, your very thoughts cause you to relax progressively more and more. As you get yourself comfortably situated in the blanket and sheets, this causes you to grow more and more relaxed. And as you place your head on the pillow and close your eyelids, this causes your subconscious mind to whisper to the brain to send you into a deep, deep natural sleep and you do sleep the entire night without disturbance, except in a case of emergency, and you do awaken at the appointed hour the next morning fully refreshed and alert.

DEPRESSION

Depression is a fine example of a way to destroy a person's physical being; for sorrow, that has no vent in tears, may make the other organs weep. When one attempts to hide or deny depression, the organs of the human body absorb the symptoms and sensations.

Depression is not a disease but a symptom tied to anxiety and fear, and continues to perpetuate itself the more the mind concentrates on it. When on a conscious level the cause is not recognized, this depressive attitude grows proportionately so that the person is unable to extricate himself.

When a person accepts depression as an escape from normal everyday events, life then becomes extremely debilitating, leading to both physical and mental deterioration. This depressive attitude is a safeguard by the person from a course of action which may be harmful due to a feeling of guilt or a need for punishment. In some cases, this need for punishment may result in suicidal tendencies. It becomes a need for a physical change to match the mental image.

All factors that cause or may cause depression must be taken into consideration, and a complete hypnoanalysis is the only choice of treatment. Some patients may continue to hold on to depressive symptoms as a means for not getting involved in what are thought to be harmful situations but, in fact, are ordinary everyday activities.

The suggestion may be as follows:

Yesterday's problems should be left with yesterday's garbage. Imagine those problems are burnt ashes and cannot be used again. Picture those ashes, the burnt problems, being discarded so those problems, once discarded, cannot cloud tomorrow's pleasures. Rejoice, for that was yesterday, a long time ago.

Assure the patient that he can be content in whatever he chooses to do. It is not what happens or doesn't happen, but how he reacts to it. I visualize everyone as being a very good hypnotic subject since he wants to be and thinks he can be; for each has been doing his own hypnosis since the day he was born so that by now, he should be an expert.

When these depressive patients are in need and there is positive motivation by the hypnotist, they will achieve their own desired depth, adequate for each and every need. Therefore, suggest that the patient need not be afraid of anything but imagine that he is doing the very thing that he fears the most and that by doing this very thing, he can realize that control is now at hand.

Remove these depressive thoughts, and replace them with positive and successful thoughts. Any insolvable problem should be left in God's hands for Him to resolve in His own way. Believing in God's infallibility allows the depression to just melt away.

Use the formula for depression.

ASTHMA

Asthma is a symptom of some underlying emotional problem and does not really exist as a disease. The initial sensitizing event, that which precipitated the first attack, does not always begin in early childhood. Fear and anxiety cause nervous tension. The greater the fear, the more tension, resulting in muscular spasm of the bronchioles. The greater the spasms, the greater the fear, and so goes this vicious cycle, resulting in the flight-or-fight syndrome.

The only thing that drugs or medication can do is relax these bronchial muscles, and this relief is only temporary. Learning to relax naturally creates the same relief. Combining this with the removal of the initial sensitizing event leads to lasting relief.

CHOKING OR GAGGING

The greater majority of gagging problems are iatrogenic in nature – that is, they are inadvertently introduced to the patient by an unintentional remark of the physician or dentist – while choking, on the one hand, is experience-related. Choking brings about a heightened sense of anxiety and increased frustration in one's inability to immediately relieve a life-threatening situation. Such anxieties create unintentional and accidental hypnosis, and coupled with the thought, *I can't breathe*, enhance the fear of swallowing and impending death. It is the fear of the food becoming lodged so that it is impossible to breathe that causes the neck muscles to respond in such a manner as to prevent the acceptance of food into that area.

Choking is a rejection of food, and this rejection is due to fear of becoming stuck. Gagging is the rejection of medical or dental instruments, trays, tongue depressors, or anything put into the mouth. To relieve one's choking problem the hypnotist impresses upon the patient, by subtle suggestions, that he possesses a throat, a neck, a mouth, teeth, and a tongue, which are all that is necessary to eat food. The suggestion may be as follows:

> Your teeth are like choppers to grind and reduce the food into small particles, allowing the tongue to move these particles to the back of the mouth, where the muscles deposit them into the chute to send them down to the stomach. You have done this thousands of times before you came here. Even when you were a small baby, you did this without any conscious effort. Now that you are older, you are more experienced and can do it much easier. Every eating experience is a new and separate event, and all prior difficulties have no effect on the next time you eat. So go ahead and create a whole new and wonderful experience by placing some very enjoyable food into your mouth. Use your choppers to break down the fibers and make such tiny pieces that they do slide down to the stomach with no conscious effort. Eating is a simple procedure, for it takes no effort at all.

To relieve gagging, suggestions may be directed as follows:

> Gagging is merely a reflex to push anything out of your mouth with the aid of your tongue. The secret for preventing gagging is to pull your tongue as far back

into your throat as possible and hold it there. Now while you are holding your tongue in this position, tap with your foot or your fingers and see how high you can count before you release your tongue from this position. I'm sure that without any effort at all, you can count almost endlessly.

When the patient is about to count beyond twenty, then continue:

Now imagine and picture that I am gently going to place in your mouth a tasty sucker (or candy, etc.), so put your tongue way back, start counting, separate your lips, and allow this nice sucker (or candy, etc.) into your mouth. Keep counting, hold your tongue back, and when I take the sucker (or candy, etc.) out, you may relax.

STUTTERING

Research has revealed a most astonishing fact: "Stuttering is primarily limited to males and not all stuttering begins with the childhood years." Stuttering is a manifestation of some inner neurosis and usually begins in childhood due to high emotional intensity. Because the etiology of this underlying neurosis consists of a child accepting a negative suggestion during a stressful period (unintentional hypnosis), its removal is brought about by intentionally returning the individual to the same state of mind. This course of stuttering usually follows one particular traumatic event of unintentional hypnosis. Consequently, every stutterer must be examined individually to determine the sensitizing events. In most cases, the onset of stuttering can readily be determined; however, it is the event that must be uncovered. Once the time has been determined, discovering the event is not so difficult.

Treatment consists of the removal of emotional disorders and the physical habits. Once the cause of the disorder is removed, the stuttering will usually disappear. During subsequent times of emotional distress, the frequency of stuttering may increase. Posthypnotic suggestion of relaxation during conversations will reduce the frequency.

Personally, I have found that the better practice is to remove all ability to speak while in a hypnotic state and then return this ability without the impediment.

Following the induction, the patient is put through the progressive relaxation and the deepening processes. Additional fast, intermittent suggestions of relaxation may also be interjected:

Each and every word I speak causes you to relax

even progressively more and more.

Each passing moment causes you to go deeper and

deeper into relaxation.

The patient should now be ready for positive responses to suggestions that the leg is numb, useless, heavy, and totally relaxed. The palm of the hand is placed on the thigh of the numb leg. Suggestions are then directed that the numb, useless, and relaxed feeling of the leg is being absorbed by the hand, acting as a sponge. The arm is then lifted, and the hand is placed on the neck of the patient.

Continue as follows:

And now all that numb, useless, and relaxed feeling

is being absorbed from the hand into the neck, causing

the neck muscles to be numb and useless.

(Gently rub the subject's hand on his neck.)

This numb and useless feeling is spreading into the

jaw muscles and lips causing them to be numb and

useless. Now this numb feeling is flowing from the lips

into the mouth, spreading that feeling deep into the mouth muscles and maybe into the tongue. Still flowing deeper and deeper into the neck, touching the vocal cords, causing them to be so numb and useless that you cannot speak one word.

I'm going to ask you some questions and you know all the answers, but as you think about these answers, your thoughts cause the numbness to penetrate deeper and deeper so you cannot speak one word. You can't even tell me your first name. Think about it and try, but you cannot .... You can't tell me what day of the week it is. Think about that .... You can't even tell me what city you live in. You can now stop trying. It's okay.

Using the formula technique, continue as follows:

In a moment, I am going to remove all impediments to your ability to speak, including those that prevented you from expressing yourself clearly and without hesitation. Recognize and realize that no one or anything is touching you or preventing you from speaking. Your thoughts alone have been holding you back.

I'm going to gently rub your forehead with my fingers and as I do so, this erases all prior thoughts that prevented you from speaking clearly ...

(Gently rub and slowly stroke the subject's forehead while the instruction continues.)

... like an eraser removing all prior impressions that you have been retaining which have prevented you from expressing yourself in words and actions. Free yourself.

Accept the fact that you can speak clearly and distinctly.
Your diction is excellent, and your enunciation is perfect.
Why, the words flow out so easily without any conscious
effort.

(Stop rubbing the subject's forehead.)

Now go ahead and tell me your name ... the day of
the week .... That's just fine. As you think about
speaking, your very thoughts cause the words to flow
right out of your mouth with ease and comfort.

FRIGIDITY AND IMPOTENCY

Frigidity and impotency are not conditions involving the
body from the waist down but from the neck up. They begin when
one is unhappy with his or her own self-concept and the acceptance
of failure of sexual satisfaction. Frigidity and impotency are socially
related and as with other difficulties, the longer the condition is
allowed to remain, the more permanent it becomes.

Treatment, therefore, must begin with the recognition of
the initial dissatisfaction and every one thereafter, including
especially the first and last.

As in most hypnotherapy, the first session is devoted to
fact finding while the patient is in a state of hypnosis. Discussion
relating to sexual conduct should include how, why, the need, for
whose benefit, the approach or foreplay, and any fears associated
with sex.

A word association test should be conducted while the
patient is in a state of hypnosis to apprise the hypnotist of the fears,
frustrations, and concerns. A list of words or phrases is prepared in
advance, and the patient is asked to listen to the word or phase and
respond by stating what enters into his or her thoughts when it is
heard.

The following words and responses are some examples:

father .... "hate"
husband .... "difficult"
sex .... "unimportant" or "important"
I don't like .... "being dominated"
I'm afraid of .... "getting pregnant"
life .... "unpleasant"
alone .... "relaxing"

Fear leads to frustration and failure is close behind. The hypnotist must very patiently but persistently delve into all of the fears associated with sexual conduct; for fear of one item alone is not sufficient to create the problem. Bring to light these fears, remove them by minimizing their importance, and reinforce the pleasures of sex.

ANESTHESIA

Suggestions of progressive relaxation should start with the eyebrows and continue down to the toes and should be conducted twice. Just before the second relaxation say:

Now we are going to do that progressive relaxation one more time, and concentrate so that you can really let yourself relax.

The second progressive relaxation permits the individual to release any residual tension and center his attention within. Relaxation does not automatically cause anesthesia so in order to create this condition, the proper suggestions are directed to the individual. The suggestions can be made to the right side as well as to the left. The following example is made to the left side:

Now just let yourself relax, just get comfortable and rested, and as you allow yourself to rest peacefully, you may experience your left leg becoming more and more relaxed, rested, comfortable. As you allow your body to continue to relax more and more, this causes your left leg to be noticeably more relaxed. From your hip all the way down to your toes, that left leg continues to grow more relaxed. Why, almost like it's falling asleep, pleasantly relaxed.

As this relaxation settles deeper and deeper into the leg, the leg seems to be getting heavier and heavier and more relaxed, limp, numb, and almost useless. From the leg all the way down to your toes, that leg becomes more relaxed, limp, rested, useless, and free of any discomfort. And that's all right.

Now I'm going to lift your left arm and place your left hand on your left thigh.

(The therapist places the subject's hand on the subject's thigh.)

Now your hand, acting like a sponge, is beginning to absorb all that numb, relaxed, and restful, useless feeling. Sponging up all that feeling from your whole leg into that tiny hand. All that feeling from your whole leg now consolidated into that little hand, causing the hand to grow progressively more relaxed, numb, useless, and limp.

Now I'm going to pick up your left arm and lift that limp, numb, and useless hand and place it on your chin.

(The therapist lifts the subject's arm and guides the hand to the chin or any other place the anesthesia is desired.)

Now this feeling from your hand starts to flow into your chin, causing your chin to become numb, limp, and useless. Growing progressively more numb as I gently rub the hand around your chin. The hand is growing perfectly normal as this feeling is being absorbed into the chin. This numb feeling now begins to spread over and into the lips, into the gums, and into all of your mouth muscles.

Any touch by a finger or instrument causes the area touched to grow progressively more and more numb. Nothing bothers you, nothing disturbs you ...

Utilizing this technique, the hypnotist may transfer the numb feeling to any part of the body. The suggestion of the touch by a finger or instrument maintains and deepens the feeling during treatment or surgery.

WEIGHT LOSS

To begin, the suggestion may be as follows:

One-half (or any other amount) of what you ordinarily eat at any regular meal is sufficient and does satisfy all of your nutritional needs and desires. The second half of what you eat causes you to maintain or put on weight, and this second half now is unacceptable to you. Everything that you know from past experiences which causes you to put on weight is now so unacceptable that it borders on the verge of being repulsive.

When you have eaten one-half of what you normally eat, you are full, stuffed, and satisfied, and this feeling of satisfaction does last from one meal to the next. Now that you are fully satisfied, you have no need or desire to eat between meals. You do now recognize that eating between meals causes you to put on weight and to maintain your weight. And that for you is entirely unacceptable, so unacceptable that the very thought of eating between meals causes a feeling of repulsiveness.

Using the formula technique, continue as follows:

Likewise, any specific food such as candy, cake, ice cream, potato chips or any other snack you now know to be unacceptable is repulsive, for it also causes you to maintain and put on weight. You do feel comfortable and satisfied without those items of food that you now know to be unacceptable.

16

SELF-HYPNOSIS

Self-hypnosis is the means by which an individual may tap into his reservoir of unlimited potential. Using self-hypnosis, subsequent to heterohypnosis, transfers the hypnotic suggestion from the hypnotist to the individual. When the suggestions become his suggestions, they are followed more readily because the desire is enhanced and the resistance is substantially reduced.

Whenever possible, the subject should learn self-hypnosis through posthypnotic suggestions. Performing self-hypnosis is akin to prescribing and receiving medication designed for a particular ailment. Although self-hypnosis is most useful in treating symptomatic problems, many organic ailments, having their origin in unintentional or accidental hypnosis, can be treated successfully.

Instructions for self-hypnosis should be kept as simple as possible and must be intellectually acceptable to the subject. Having previously experienced hypnotic inductions, the subject should be taught self-hypnosis using induction methods similar to those already employed by the hypnotist. While the subject is in a state of hypnosis, the following language may be used to teach self-hypnosis:

> You know that each and every time I suggest
> relaxation, you do relax. Each and every time I suggest
> relaxation, this causes your eyes to grow tired and
> causes your eyelids to grow heavy. So when I then lower
> my hand down closer to your forehead, this causes your
> eyes to grow progressively more and more tired and your
> eyelids to grow heavy ... progressively more and more

heavy. And you know that before my hand touches your forehead, your eyelids do close and you do relax.

Each subsequent time that you relax, you do relax quicker and deeper than the previous time. Each and every time that you put your hands up above your head, you are asking your subconscious mind to relax you, just like you are now relaxing. As you lower your hands down closer and closer to your eyes, this causes your eyes to become progressively more tired and your eyelids to become progressively more and more heavy and before your hands touch your forehead, your eyelids do close and you do relax, just like you are now relaxed.

I am going to reach down and pick up your hands gently by the wrists and put them in the position that I am talking about.

Reach for the wrists and gently lift the hands up about a foot above the forehead, palms down. You may put one hand over the other so that only one palm is shown.

Continue as follows:

Each and every time you place your hands in this position, you are asking your subconscious mind to relax your whole body. Still remaining deeply relaxed, open your eyes and look into the palm of your hand.

(The subject opens his eyes and looks up into the palm.)

By looking into the palm of your hand, your subconscious mind recognizes and realizes your need and desire to go into a deep state of relaxation. Now as you slowly lower your hands, this causes your eyes to become progressively more tired and your eyelids more and more heavy.

(Still holding the hands, now slowly guide them down to the eyes.)

And before your hands touch your forehead, your eyelids close and you do relax.

(The eyelids of the subject close. Let go of the subject's hands when they touch the forehead.)

Now put your hands in any position that you feel most comfortable. This is the first step of self-hypnosis, and it is called the induction. Realize that all you are doing is entering into a state of relaxation.

The next step is to deepen this state of relaxation.

Concentrate or focus your attention on your eyelids and create a feeling in your eyelids and your eye muscles that for you is comfortable, pleasant, peaceful, restful, and relaxing. Hold your direction and attention on your eyelids and eye muscles, and create a feeling of total and complete relaxation just as much as you can. Stay with your eyelids and eye muscles. Really relax those eyelids and eye muscles.

Now you direct your attention to the area around your forehead and your eyebrows. You think about the skin on the forehead, and you make your skin nice and soft.

Get the skin smooth and comfortable. If you can, picture and imagine that right on the center of the forehead, you have a nice spot, a dab of creamy, fluffy

lotion sitting right on the center of the forehead, just
above the bridge of your nose. Lotion that you know
from past experience is comfortable, lotion that is
pleasant, and lotion that penetrates, seeping into the
tiny pores of your skin.

So imagine this lotion slowly beginning to absorb the
warmth of your body and slowly beginning to spread
and flowing across your forehead, soothing, penetrating,
comforting, relaxing all the way across your forehead.
Then imagine that this pleasant feeling of comfort,
slowly trickles and flows from the forehead down over
and across your temples and down into your cheeks.

Now you think about your cheeks and you relax
your cheeks. Make your cheek muscles nice and limp and
loose and rested and relaxed. Give the cheek muscles the
sensation, the symptom that they want to melt a little
bit, trying to let go but still kind of stuck there and
growing pleasantly more limp, loose, and rested. And
you find that each passing moment causes your cheek
muscles and your eyelids and eye muscles to relax
progressively more.

So now while your cheek muscles continue to relax
even more and more, allow some of this relaxation from
your cheeks down into your jaw muscles, deep in the jaw
muscles. Let the jaw muscles just go limp, loose, and
relaxed. And then spread this relaxation over to your
chin and over to your lips.

Now you think about your lips, and you relax those lips of yours. Make your lips nice and soft and tender, soothing, comfortable, restful, and relaxing. So you think about your lips, and let all the muscles in your lips and your mouth muscles relax.

So go ahead, relax everything as much as you can. Relax the jaw muscles, the chin, the cheek muscles, the lips. You see, as you relax all these muscles, your lips have a tendency to part and separate pleasantly and comfortably as this relaxation penetrates even deeper and deeper.

And from the forehead imagine something soothing, something comfortable, something very pleasant slowly flowing and spreading from your forehead up across the top of the head. Soothing and caressing the top of the head, penetrating deep, deep inside, sending a feeling of comfort deep within.

Imagine this sensation of comfort spreads all the way across the top of your head and the pleasant feeling flows and trickles down the back of your head, soothing and caressing the back of the head. Let this wonderful feeling slowly settle deep into the back of the neck muscles. So you think about all these areas, and relax each and every one of these areas.

Now imagine you can experience the sensation, the feeling that this relaxation has a tendency to become loose and the pleasant feeling of relaxation seems to drain down from the top of the head, flow down from the forehead and the eyelids, slowly drain down from the cheeks, seep down from the lips, down through the neck and down to your shoulders, and slowly flow and spread across your shoulders, touching, soothing, comforting all the shoulder muscles.

So now you think about the shoulder muscles. You think about the large and the small muscles in your shoulders and allow your shoulder muscles to become just totally limp and completely relaxed. Let the shoulder muscles kind of sag and hang a little bit. Just let go. Just let go. Imagine that this wonderful, soothing feeling of relaxation spreads all the way across your shoulders, and now something soothing and comfortable, pleasant and peaceful, flows over your shoulders, down both of your arms.

Imagine something so pleasant, so comfortable, so restful and relaxing, flowing down both of your arms, not only over the skin but deep, deep inside. Imagine the sensation of relaxation slowly flowing downward, downward, touching, penetrating, soothing, and caressing all the muscles in both of your arms, resting and relaxing each and every nerve, all the tendons, the fibers, touching and soothing and comforting every tissue in every cell, everything from the shoulders down to your elbows.

Now you think about your arms from the elbows to your shoulders, and you let your arms become pleasantly and comfortably and deeply relaxed. As you relax your arms from the shoulders to the elbows, this causes your body to relax from the shoulders down to the hips, growing progressively more and more relaxed. And now this relaxation continues to flow down past the elbows again over the skin and deep inside your arms, soothing, comforting all the muscles in both of your arms. Even caressing all of the nerves, tendons, and tissues. Relaxing every cell, every gland and every fiber. Everything from the elbows all the way down to your wrist. As you relax your arms from the shoulders to the wrists this causes your body to relax from the shoulders down to your hips, past your hips and down to your toes.

Now imagine this relaxation continues to flow down past the wrist. Imagine something so pleasant, so comfortable slowly flowing from the wrists over the back of both of your hands, and a soothing sensation spreads down into the palms of both of your hands. Now all of this relaxation continues to flow down into each and every one of your fingers, causing your arms from the shoulders down to the finger tips to grow progressively more and more relaxed. As you allow your arms to relax from the shoulders past the elbows and down to your finger tips, this causes your whole body to relax from the top of your head down to your shoulders, past your hips, and all the way down to your toes.

Each passing moment causes your body to relax
progressively more and more. Then imagine this
relaxation slowly beginning to flow from your shoulders
down your chest and down your back. Imagine your
body being covered, even draped if you like, in the most
restful, the most comfortable, the most soothing, the
most peaceful sensation you could ever experience.
Slowly flowing from the shoulders, down to the chest
area, penetrating deep in the chest, spreading all the
way across the chest, even down the sides of your body.

Now from the back of the shoulders, imagine a
soothing sensation slowly trickling down through the
back muscles, penetrating, resting, relaxing all of the
back muscles, flowing all the way down, down into the
lower back. From the chest area the sensation of
relaxation spreads down and flows into the stomach
area. Then all this relaxation continues to flow, slowly,
down into the hips, momentarily stopping at the hips,
but spreading all the way across the hips, penetrating
deep, deep in those hips, touching and soothing and
caressing all of the muscles, each and every tendon and
every nerve and every cell in those hips of yours.

Now as you spread this relaxation from your hips
down to your thighs, it's time for you to picture and
imagine you are in your comfort zone, your sanctuary,
the place where you go to be alone with your thoughts.
Just think about a place where you could be alone,
undisturbed, just with your own thoughts.

If the library was used during the first session (and other sessions) and the subject's responses were satisfactory, then return the subject back to the library. However, if the therapist was not satisfied with the subject's responses or if the subject was not entirely comfortable with the library, then another place may be suggested.

I'm not sure you were very comfortable in the library so if you would like to go to another place, it is perfectly all right. Some people like to go to the beach and walk or sit on the sand and enjoy the nice warm fresh air. Some like to walk ankle deep in the water along the beach and look out over the water and see a ship or a sailboat not too far away.

Last week a gentleman preferred to sit in a large room with a big fireplace and watch the multicolored dancing flames and feel the warmth of the fireplace and hear the sound of a crackling log. I had a woman in today that said she liked to go for a walk in the woods, smell the fresh air, listen to the breeze as it rustles the branches, look up and see the sunlight as it glistens through the leaves, listen to a bird and an animal scamper not too far away. A gentleman preferred to sit on the side of a small mountain and look over the valley. It gave him a feeling of being away from everything.

So maybe you would like to go some place I have suggested or some place where you have been before or a place you can just imagine. So I will give you a little time to select your sanctuary, your comfort area. When

you have selected such a place, just nod your head YES
so I know that you have made a selection.

(The subject nods his head "yes.")

When the head has nodded "yes," then the therapist should
ask the subject to share with him the place that has been selected.
Now the therapist should ask the subject to describe the area, one
part of the picture at a time. For example, should a beach scene be
selected, the subject may be asked:

Is there any seaweed or shells around? Can you
smell the seawater in the air? Has the water washed up
any debris on the sand? Are there any birds soaring with
the wind?

If the fireplace scene was selected, these questions may be
asked:

Do you hear any crackling of the logs? Are there
any other logs that can be placed on the fire? Are you
sitting on a chair or lying on the floor? Can you feel the
warmth of the fire?

The subject may select a path in the woods, then you can ask:

Can you see the rays of the sun filter through the
branches? Are there any pine cones around? In your
absence, did anyone leave any cans or paper in retreat?
Can you hear the wind rustling the leaves?

Continue as follows:

Each and every time you go to your comfort zone,
your sanctuary, your retreat, the picture gets clearer and
clearer.

Now it is time for your suggestive therapy. And what are you going to think about? You are going to think about your needs and your desires, the changes you want to make in your life. Your thoughts must follow, and I repeat, must follow a particular and prescribed formula.

First of all, the word will should never be used in your suggestive therapy. The word will means something is going to happen in the future. You only function in the present time, at this very moment. So all of our suggestions must be in the present tense. You see, everything for you begins now and continues into the future.

You are going to think about two things: one is those events that you wish to create or those events that you wish to discard and eliminate, and the second is how you feel participating in the new events and how you feel not doing the things that you used to do. The second is equally important as the first. So get yourself comfortable in your sanctuary, your comfort zone, your retreat. You can either sit down in a comfortable position or walk about.

Imagine that in this position you are now the person you want to be (that is, characteristically or personality-wise) and that now you do all the things you desire to do and you feel like you like to feel at any time or place and under any and all circumstances. Imagine you are not who you used to be but are now someone different.

Now it is time for you to do some serious thinking. You think about your needs and you think about your desires. You think about the changes in life you have to make. Now you understand that everything you do in life is preceded by a thought. All your emotions and feelings, symptoms and fantasies are also preceded by a thought. And these thoughts are messages to the brain to create the condition that you think about, to create the symptom and feeling you have a need for.

You see, the brain runs your whole body. But the brain doesn't do anything until it's asked and told to do something. You've had that experience. Before you get out of a chair to walk, first you think about it. And once you make a decision to do something, the brain activates your walking program. It moves the muscles necessary to carry out and fulfill your thoughts. That's what it does. Makes things happen after the thought.

And if you're walking across a room and you see something on the floor, you may walk right past that thing on the floor. But then you decide to pick up the thing, whatever it may be. The moment you make that decision, you turn around, walk over to the object, bend over, reach out, extend your fingers, grasp the object, stand up, and place the object where you have decided to put it. You see, everything happens after you made the decision to pick up this object. And all the brain is doing is carrying out and fulfilling your desires, your messages. If you never thought about picking up the object, you'd keep right on going.

So you sit there in a nice comfortable environment and you tell yourself who you are. And if you want to be, you tell yourself, "I am the most relaxed person in the whole world. How relaxed? So relaxed that nothing bothers me. Nothing disturbs me. Nobody steals my time, my energy, my efforts. Nobody controls me. I'm in charge. Of what? I'm in charge of everything I do, everything I think about, and I'm in charge of all my emotions, my symptoms, and my fantasies. And I sure love who I am, 'cause I think I'm terrific and great."

You see, what you're doing is, you're sending all kinds of messages to the brain and the subconscious might say, "Brain, guess what message we got? And we have to fulfill and carry out every one of these directions, these thoughts, these instructions."

So if you don't send a message, you get no response. The response comes after the message. So if you want to be, you tell yourself, "I'm compassionate. I'm a caring person. I'm a lovable person, joyful and happy. I think life is terrific. I'm competent and capable. I'm a successful person. Whenever I decide to do something, I do everything I decide to do with ease and with comfort, completely relaxed. I do everything on time, no delays."

You see, you're sending messages.

322 MEDICINE OF THE MIND   DR. MICHAEL D. PRESTON

Your brain is a depository of these messages and the
brain is a processor and programmer of these messages.

Every person should be put through the same steps in the
hypnotic session. In self-hypnosis, as a post-hypnotic technique,
the hypnotist goes through the induction, progressive relaxation,
and right to the place where the suggestive therapy is conducted.
The same is true for the initial session. The therapist goes through
an induction technique, progressive relaxation, a deepening
technique, another deepening technique (counting backwards from
100 and then the classroom). The subject is then taken into the
library where the therapy is to be conducted. Having tested the
person at the initial session, there is no need to test further unless
the person exhibits some visible anxiety

As long as the therapist repeatedly states, "Each and every
time you relax, you do relax quicker and deeper than the previous
time," subsequent sessions should cause the person to be in a deep
state of hypnosis. In the event that the person does exhibit some anxiety
at any session, then another deepening technique is appropriate.

In all hypnotic sessions, the therapist must address two
things: (1) the event to be created or the event that must be
eliminated and (2) the subject must be comfortable not doing the
things he used to do, or must be comfortable doing the things he
desires to do. Unless the person is comfortable not doing the things
(smoking, drugs, excessive eating, etc.) he will return to that conduct
to bring about a relief that he does not now have. Unless so
addressed, the session is doomed to fail.

To complete this self-hypnosis session, we will continue
the therapy for a smoking cessation. Continue as follows:

I have no need and no desire for cigarettes,

chemicals wrapped in white paper. The very thought of

me putting cigarettes into my mouth with the intention

of smoking the cigarettes causes me to feel nauseated, uncomfortable, and upset; for I find smoking cigarettes unacceptable, intolerable, and totally repulsive. I don't put repulsive material in my mouth. I do feel totally uncomfortable and repulsed by smoking cigarettes. The very thought of putting cigarettes in my mouth thoroughly upsets me.

Each and every thought and word rejecting smoking causes me to feel comfortable, pleasant, and relaxed. Such words and thoughts as "I don't smoke," "I'm a non-smoker," "I'm not so foolish as to put cigarettes in my mouth," cause me to feel absolutely pleasant and relaxed.

Be creative in forming your suggestions as may be appropriate for each subject that you work with.

Continue as follows:

Now it is time for you to return to the conscious state. When you have finished your suggestive therapy (that's the thought you express and create in your comfort zone, your sanctuary) all you need to do is count from one to three and at the count of three, your eyes do open and you are alert back in your conscious state, feeling pleasant and relaxed.

Repetition in reminding the person he now has no need for his problem is helpful in disposing of these symptoms or difficulties. Depth perception by the subconscious mind is very real or when reference is made to any need or desire, acceptance of these suggestions is readily recorded within.

Suggestions, coupled with imagery, produce beneficial results. While the subject is imagining the scenery of the retreat or sanctuary, develop within this scene objects that clutter up the peaceful scene, things such as beer or soda cans, paper, cigarette packages, poorly formed pine cones, broken seashells, rotted pieces of wood, broken glass, or any item that may be considered debris. Since it is the obligation or duty of the subject to keep the sanctuary clean, these things must be picked up and discarded. However, before discarding them, a new and different identity is given to them. These items of debris can be called "hate," "anger," "pain," "old needs," "old desires," or any other symptom or problem that should be removed. The suggestions may run along these lines:

You have an obligation to keep your retreat or sanctuary free of junk, debris, or garbage. Look around, and should you find anything that doesn't belong there, just nod your head to let me know that you have found this thing.

(The subject nods his head.)

Go over to it and pick it up and hold it in your hands, and when you have it, just nod your head to let me know that you have it.

(The subject nods his head.)

Look at it and we are now going to give it a different identity. As you hold it, say to yourself, "This is my fear."

(The word "fear" may be replaced with hate, anger, depression, old need, old desires, etc.)

Take that fear and throw it into the water just as far as you can and watch it disappear. It is gone out of your life, and it can no longer disturb or bother you. So feel

good about it. Enjoy your freedom from it. Look around
and let me know when you have found some other
debris.

(The subject nods his head.)

Why don't you call this your addiction and then cast it
away into the water and watch your addiction disappear?

Regardless of the scene that the subject may develop, there
are things that can be assigned a symptom or problem. In the
fireplace scene, the logs next to the fireplace can be given an identity
and by placing the logs in the fireplace, the subject is burning away
the unwanted symptoms and problems. The subject may imagine
being in the woods near a small stream. Suggest that the subject
stand in the stream barefooted and allow the cool water to wash
away his difficulties and problems, just like being baptized and
born again. Pine cones that are deformed can be buried, which
resembles burying unwanted symptoms. Beautiful things can be
gathered and built into a monument. Beautiful seashells and various
colored rocks can be piled up, representing a castle of success and
happiness. Anything can be given an identity which represents good
or bad things. Cast away or bury the difficulties or problems and
keep those that represent the new and desired symptoms.

During the first week following the session in which self-
hypnosis is taught, the person should practice the self-hypnosis at
least five times a day; the next week he should reduce the number
of sessions each day thereafter. Many persons may express concern
about not having the time to do this five times a day However,
when they are assured that each self-hypnosis session can be
performed in just a matter of three minutes, allowing fifteen minutes
for all the benefits that can be developed, that answers most of the
objections. Self-hypnosis should be taught to each and every subject
regardless of the nature of the problems.

CONCLUSION

The subconscious mind is that path by which we travel to all other conscious entities in the entire universe. These subconscious minds of all individuals are the connecting links that provide the basis for all understanding. We are all a very important part of this mass of intelligence, for there is but one mind of the entire universe, one intelligence, and one presence.

All things are already in creation in some way and are brought into being by the intelligence of the subconscious mind. Each of us, by using the full potential of our collective minds, can find our relationship to God and to the universe which is waiting to be uncovered.

The recognition that I am presence, the awareness of the divine nature of man, is the key to the unraveling of that which is hidden.

INDEX

ABOUT THE AUTHOR

Michael D. Preston, J.D., Ph.D., first became familiar with hypnosis at the 5th Army Rehabilitation Center in Sorento, Italy, while serving in the U.S. Armed Services.

In 1947, he studied psychology and hypnotherapy with Lewis R. Wolberg, M.D., a clinical professor of psychiatry and chairman of the board at New York Medical College. From there, Dr. Preston went to Chicago, then to Los Angeles, working for the Veterans Administration.

By 1960, he was made a staff member of the American College of Medical Hypnotists; conducted seminars in the U.S. and Europe with William J. Bryan, Jr., M.D., Ph.D.; wrote and edited for the *Journal of the American Institute of Hypnosis.*

He then founded the Institute of Medical Hypnosis in Chicago in 1966. Later, he moved his practice to Phoenix, Arizona, and with the assistance of William McGrath, M.D., Dr. Preston used hypnosis to treat not only emotional and physical problems, but to treat the terminally ill patients by applying the theory of psychoneuroimmunology.

Presently, the author is affiliated with the National Society of Hypnotists, the International Society for Investigative and Forensic Hypnosis, the National Board for Hypnotherapy and Hypnotic Anesthesiology, the American Association of Behavioral Therapists, the National Guild of Hypnotists, and the Center for Advancement in Cancer Education. Dr. Preston, also known as the "Miracle Doctor," has conducted seminars in over 40 cities in the United States, Canada, and England.

The author is the recipient of the President's Award from the Florida Association of Professional Hypnotists, the Pen and Quill Award from the American Academy of Medical Hypnoanalysts; the Hypnotherapy Educator Award from the National Board for Hypnotherapy and Hypnotic Anesthesiology; and the Founder's Award from the National Board for Hypnotherapy and Hypnotic Anesthesiology.

TO ORDER VIDEO AND AUDIO TAPES

Please call or e-mail for prices and availability.
E-mail: medhypno@cs.com
Web: www.medhypno.com
Toll-free: 1-800-861-7899

SEMINAR VIDEO TAPES

The Institute of Medical Hypnosis has professionally video taped the Preston three-day Medical Hypnosis Seminar on nine (9) VHS tapes and they are now available for purchase. These informative tapes cover eighteen (18) hours of intense, detailed material, with complete informative material necessary to provide the therapist with the complete information on how to successfully treat most emotional and physical problems.

Seminar Objectives and Benefits:
- To focus on the true nature of hypnosis and the positive utilization of hypnotherapy.
- To teach the basic, advanced, and specialized inductions and deepening techniques so the patient can enter into a very deep state of hypnosis to achieve the desired results.
- To easily identify, remove, and control the causes of smoking, overweight, stress, fear, pain, anxiety, phobia, and other emotional problems.
- To teach other methods and techniques so the patient can be successfully treated.
- To teach methods and techniques to treat alcohol and drug abuse.

- To teach psychoneuroimmunology and how the state of mind, in hypnosis, can influence the immune system's fight against diseases, illness, and physical damages.
- To teach self-hypnosis and give the patient tools to continue the treatment to overcome additional problems.

AUDIO TAPES

- Enhance the Immune System to Fight: Cancer, Tourette's Syndrome, Cholesterol, Dysfunctional Kidneys, AIDS, Genital Herpes, High Blood Pressure, Tumors
- Learn to Control: Weight, Smoking, Anger, Stress, Nail Biting, Insomnia, Stress, Depression, Relationship Issues, Public Speaking, Sports, Activities, Test Passing, Guilt, Pain, Anxiety
- Learn Self-Hypnosis

4280342

Made in the USA
Lexington, KY
10 January 2010